Heart-Brain Diet

Essential Nutrition for Healthy Longevity

2020 Report

A Special Report published by the editors of
Tufts Health & Nutrition Letter
in cooperation with
The Friedman School of Nutrition Science and Policy
Tufts University

Heart-Brain Diet: Essential Nutrition for Healthy Longevity

Consulting Editor: Tammy Scott, PhD, Assistant Professor, Friedman School of Nutrition Science and Policy, Tufts University

Consulting Dietitian: Helen Rasmussen, PhD, RD, FADA, senior research dietitian, Jean Mayer USDA Human Nutrition Research Center on Aging at Tufts University

Dietetic Intern: Melissa Townsend, MS, Frances Stern Nutrition Center, Friedman School of Nutrition Science and Policy, Tufts University

Author: Stephanie Watson
Update author: David Fryxell
Creative Director, Belvoir Media Group: Judi Crouse
Belvoir Editor: Dawn Bialy
Production: Mary Francis McGavic

Publisher, Belvoir Media Group: Timothy H. Cole
Executive Editor, Book Division, Belvoir Media Group: Lynn Russo Whylly

ISBN 978-1-879620-98-8

To order additional copies of this report or for customer service questions, please call 877-300-0253, or write to Health Special Reports, 535 Connecticut Avenue, Norwalk, CT 06854-1713.

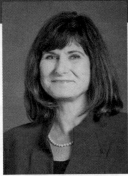

Tammy Scott, PhD
Assistant Professor,
Friedman School of
Nutrition Science
and Policy, Tufts
University

Dear Friends,

Centuries before the breakthroughs achieved by modern medicine, medieval philosophers believed the human heart was "the root of all faculties"—the source of what makes each person unique. Though we now understand that cognition and consciousness spring instead from the brain, those ancient thinkers were not far wrong in emphasizing the central role of the heart. Today, research is increasingly demonstrating that what's good for your heart is also good for your brain. That is the core message of this book and the basis of its dietary and lifestyle recommendations.

This crucial heart-brain connection begins with the circulatory system. Studies have shown that adults with the highest levels of cardiovascular fitness are the least likely to die of dementia, while those with cardiovascular disease also are more likely to suffer brain impairments and dementia. We also know that people with a greater volume of blood flow from the heart also tend to have a larger brain volume.

What You Can Do. The associations between heart and brain health also extend to nutrition. Many of the same nutrients that benefit the heart and vascular system are essential to the brain. When you adopt a heart-healthy dietary pattern, those nutritional choices benefit your brain as well.

This is especially good news given the frustrating lack of progress of research on Alzheimer's disease. Alzheimer's and other forms of dementia can be frightening, and, as yet, scientists have found no medical prevention or cure for these debilitating diseases. Nonetheless, we can take heart—literally—in knowing that a heart-healthy diet and lifestyle can make a difference. While you are reducing the odds of cognitive decline and dementia, you also are protecting yourself against cardiovascular disease.

Dietary Recommendations. Science-based nutritional guidance for both your heart and brain is integral to the missions of Tufts University's Friedman School of Nutrition Science and Policy and Jean Mayer USDA Human Nutrition Research Center on Aging. Our research explores ways in which dietary patterns, as well as specific foods and nutrients, can improve your cardiovascular health and reduce your risk of cognitive decline and dementia. In this publication, we share important findings from Tufts and other research institutions throughout the world that have advanced our understanding of how nutrition affects your heart and brain.

Also in these pages, you will find specific recipes to help you take steps toward adopting a diet that's optimal for your heart and brain. As you will see, eating right for your heart and brain can be easy as well as delicious.

We may now know that the heart is not actually "the root of all faculties," but it is vital to the functioning of the brain that makes you uniquely you. By taking steps now to protect your heart and brain, you are investing in a future in which you can live healthier longer.

Sincerely,

Tammy Scott, PhD

Tammy Scott, PhD

TABLE OF CONTENTS

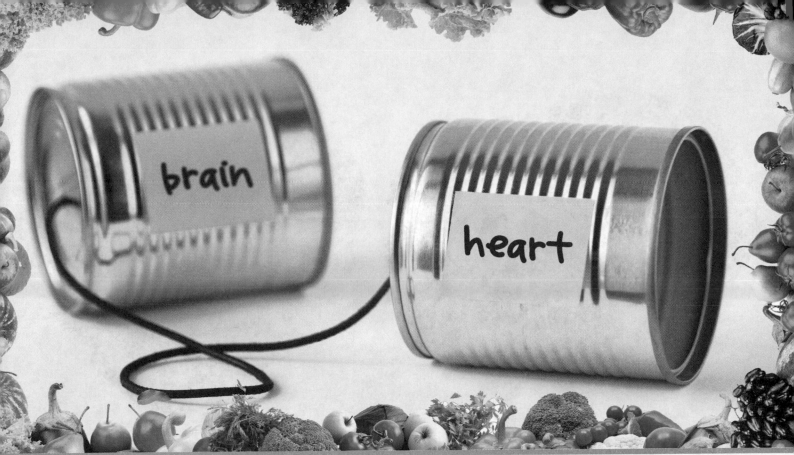

New Findings

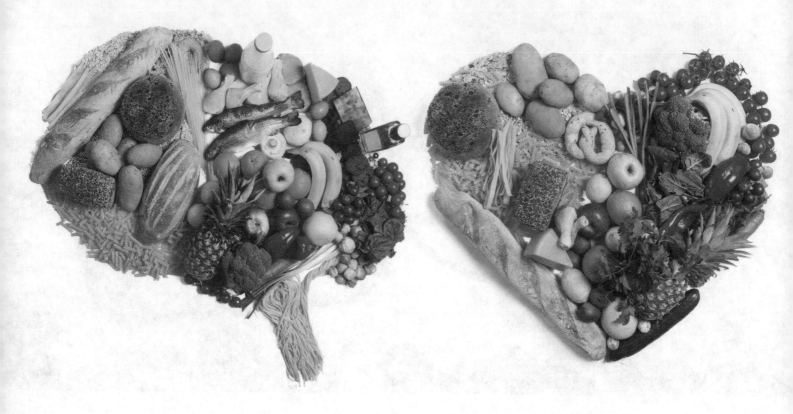

Your circulatory system, which is driven by your heart, supplies your brain with the oxygen and nutrients it needs. Your heart, blood vessels, and brain all benefit from a healthy diet.

1 The Heart-Brain Connection

You may be wondering why this book is titled *Heart-Brain Diet*. After all, your heart and brain are very different organs with entirely different functions. At the most basic level, one organ employs muscle to pump blood throughout the body, while the other is a mass of tissue through which electrical impulses flow. But these two organs are deeply interconnected, which is why a dietary pattern that benefits one also helps protect the other.

Though your heart and cardiovascular system have many functions, none is more important than keeping your brain supplied with energy and oxygen. Biologically speaking, that organ inside your skull is kept alive by the beating of an organ in your chest. To supply blood to the brain and the body's other organs, your heart beats about 100,000 times a day, pumping 2,000 gallons of blood through more than 60,000 miles of blood vessels.

And the brain is quite demanding: Although an average brain makes up only about two percent of total body weight, it consumes 20 percent of the energy from food you eat and 20 percent of the oxygen you breathe. Under ordinary circumstances, your brain uses 20 to 25 percent of the blood supply circulated by your heart. When your brain is hard at work, it requires even more blood.

A 2018 study provided evidence of the link between a healthy heart and a healthy brain. In the study, women who scored the highest on a test of cardiovascular fitness were 88 percent less likely to develop dementia than women with average scores on the fitness test, while those with the lowest fitness scores were at 41 percent greater risk of dementia.

Lifestyle Changes Pay Off

If you have a family history of cardiovascular disease or dementia, you may be wondering if it's worth making dietary and lifestyle changes to protect your heart and your brain. Genetics certainly play a role, but your genes are not your destiny. Research suggests a healthy lifestyle may cut the risk of heart disease events (such as heart attack) by about half.

In one study, scientists looked at genetic and medical data from four studies involving more than 50,000 adults. They assessed lifestyle using four criteria: avoiding obesity, following a heart-healthy dietary pattern, exercising at least once a week, and no current smoking. Meeting at least three of the four favorable lifestyle criteria was associated with a 46 percent reduction in risk of heart events compared to meeting only one or none of the healthy lifestyle criteria—and this held true regardless of genetic risk. On the other hand, meeting one or none of the four criteria reduced the protective effects associated with low genetic risk by about half.

These findings also suggest that diet and lifestyle changes can benefit your brain, whatever your genetic predisposition. A growing body of research indicates that a diet that supports a healthy heart is also brain-healthy fare and vice versa. Learning which foods your heart and brain need to function optimally and how to incorporate these foods into an everyday eating plan can help protect both of these vital organs.

That's the mission of this book: To provide you with information and strategies that you can use to reduce your risks of developing diseases of the heart and brain.

The Circulatory System and Your Brain

Your body is constantly circulating more than five quarts of blood; to keep that blood moving, your heart will beat more than 2.5 billion times during an average lifetime. Of course, the job of keeping your brain supplied with blood and nutrients doesn't end with your heart. Even if your heart is healthy and doing its job, your brain also relies on blood vessels that provide it with nutrients and oxygen: Whatever is bad for these blood vessels is bad for your brain.

In one study, for example, participants who had a higher risk of vascular disease due to blood pressure, diabetes, and smoking had a greater chance of later developing dementia. Diabetes was associated with a 77 percent higher dementia risk; a 41 percent higher risk was linked to smoking and a 39 percent higher risk was linked to hypertension.

Vascular dementia, the second most common form of dementia after Alzheimer's disease, is one clear example of the damage your brain can suffer if there are problems in your circulatory system. Vascular dementia is caused by a stroke or a series of tiny strokes that cut off or restrict the flow of blood to brain cells. Narrowing and stiffness of blood vessels also can accelerate cognitive decline, as well as the degree of impairment that occurs due to Alzheimer's disease or a condition known as dementia with Lewy bodies (also called Lewy body dementia).

It's not just the blood vessels directly supplying the brain that are important, however. In another study, researchers measured levels of calcified plaque in participants' coronary arteries—the blood vessels that feed the heart. Seven years later, participants took a battery of cognitive tests. Those who had more plaque in their arteries initially had poorer cognitive function later.

Understanding Blood Flow

The number-one job of the circulatory system is to keep your blood flowing. Your blood is made up of plasma, red

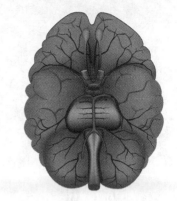

Arteries in the Brain

Arteries supply your brain with nutrients and oxygen.

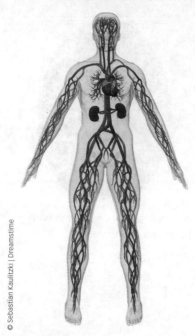

Your circulatory system is a network of arteries (in red, above), veins (in blue, above), and capillaries, the tiny blood vessels through which oxygen, nutrients, and waste products are exchanged.

© Sebastian Kaulitzki | Dreamstime

blood cells, platelets, and white blood cells. Plasma contains substances involved in blood clotting. Red blood cells transport oxygen using a substance called hemoglobin that binds to oxygen in your lungs. Platelets cause your blood to form clots to stop bleeding, and white blood cells defend against infection.

In a process that repeats itself as long as your heart keeps beating, the circulatory system delivers oxygen-depleted blood to the right atrium, one of two upper chambers in the heart. Blood then flows to the right ventricle, which pumps blood to the lungs to pick up a fresh batch of oxygen. Oxygen-rich blood is then received by the left atrium and transferred to the left ventricle, which pushes it out through the aorta. Once the brain or other parts of the body extract the oxygen, the cycle starts all over again, with the depleted blood arriving in the right atrium to be replenished.

Paths for Blood Flow

The body utilizes two primary pathways for blood flow. The part of the circulatory system that serves the brain, the heart, and most of the rest of the body is called "systemic circulation." The other pathway serves the lungs (pulmonary circulation). Carrying the blood through this network is a system of blood vessels consisting of arteries, veins, and capillaries. In this network, the arteries and veins are the main roads, and the capillaries are the side streets. In addition to supplying the body with oxygen, this system also transports nutrients and waste products.

Arteries such as the aorta, which is the largest artery, carry oxygen-rich blood from the heart to the rest of the body. As the arteries branch off farther away from the heart, they get smaller. Arteries carry large amounts of blood under a high amount of pressure from the heart. Muscles in these walls continually squeeze to keep the blood moving

smoothly. The arteries are lined with an inside layer, the endothelium, that provides a smooth surface over which the blood can easily flow.

Once the body's tissues and organs have received oxygen and nutrients from the bloodstream, the depleted blood is brought back to the heart by veins. The largest vein in your body is the inferior vena cava, which returns blood from the lower half of your body to your heart.

The tiny blood vessels that supply the body's tissues and organs are the capillaries. Capillaries have thin walls that enable oxygen, nutrients, and carbon dioxide to pass easily to and from the body's cells.

Protecting the Brain

The brain is protected by a special checkpoint called the blood-brain barrier. This barrier is a semi-permeable system that allows only certain substances to pass into the brain—unlike other parts of the systemic circulatory network, in which nutrients, oxygen, and waste products can move freely in and out of the capillaries. The blood-brain barrier protects the brain against viruses, toxins, and other substances in the blood that might harm the brain's delicate tissues. The blood-brain barrier also prevents many compounds you might take in supplement form from reaching the brain; this means you should be skeptical of pills that promise cognitive benefits through direct action on your brain. (An exception is melatonin, which can cross the blood-brain barrier.)

The circulatory system transports blood to the brain through the carotid arteries, located on either side of the neck, and the vertebral arteries, which extend alongside the spinal column in the back of the neck.

When Things Go Wrong

Problems can arise in the heart and elsewhere in the circulatory system, just as they can in any of the body's systems. These problems have implications for the brain as well. The most common cardiovascular problems are explained briefly below.

Arrhythmia

When the electrical impulses inside the heart that control the heartbeat get out of rhythm, the heart can beat erratically, too quickly, or too slowly. This irregular heart rhythm is called an arrhythmia. A severe arrhythmia can impair the heart's ability to pump enough blood through-out the body.

Atherosclerosis

When plaque deposits made up of fat, cholesterol, and other substances build up on artery walls, the result is athero-sclerosis, or "hardening of the arteries." Over time, this plaque buildup stiffens arteries and can narrow or completely block them. These narrowed arteries can develop clots that block blood flow, and bits of plaque can break off and block smaller arteries. Such blockages are a common cause of cardiovascular events such as stroke and heart attack.

Atrial Fibrillation

Known as "A-fib" for short, atrial fibril-lation happens when an irregular heart-beat occurs in the two upper chambers of the heart (the atria). Atrial fibrillation is especially relevant to brain health because it can cause blood to pool and form a clot that can travel to the brain, blocking a blood vessel and causing a stroke. Having atrial fibrillation can raise your stroke risk by as much as five times.

Carotid Artery Disease

The carotid arteries that feed the front part of the brain also are susceptible to plaque buildup, causing carotid artery disease. If the blood flow in a carotid artery is blocked by plaque, it can damage or destroy brain cells. Carotid artery disease can lead to a stroke or a transient ischemic attack (TIA), also called a "mini-stroke."

Coronary Artery Disease

Similarly, when plaque accumulates in the arteries that supply blood, oxygen, and nutrients to the heart, it causes a condition called coronary artery disease (or coronary heart disease). Coronary artery disease is the most common heart condition in adults. When plaque builds up on walls of the coronary arteries, the artery narrows and decreases the blood flow to the heart. Complete blockage of an artery may cause a heart attack (myo-cardial infarction), and the section of the heart tissue that is starved of oxygen may be permanently damaged. Plaque buildup also can lead to the formation of clots; a heart attack may result if a clot breaks free and blocks a blood ves-sel in the heart.

Stroke

The most common type of stroke, an ischemic stroke, occurs as a result of an obstruction within an artery that sup-plies blood to the brain or is in the brain itself. Ischemic strokes account for about 87 percent of all strokes. The obstruc-tions can take two forms:

- A blood clot (thrombus) that develops in an artery within the brain is a cerebral thrombosis.
- A blood clot that forms elsewhere, most often in the heart or the large arteries of the upper chest and neck, breaks loose into the bloodstream and travels into the brain until it blocks a smaller blood vessel; this is called a cerebral embolism.

The second major type of stroke, hemorrhagic stroke, results from weak-ened blood vessels in the brain that rupture and bleed. The accumulated blood can damage the surrounding brain tissue.

Damage Caused by Blood Clots

HEART ATTACK

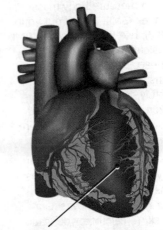

Blood clot blocks blood flow to the heart muscle

STROKE

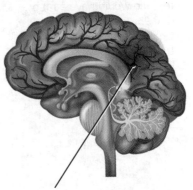

Blood clot blocks blood flow to or in the brain

© Guniita | Dreamstime

In addition to the brain damage that may be caused by a stroke, victims of stroke who survive are at greater risk of impaired cognitive function. One study found that stroke survivors experienced a 23 percent relative acceleration in cognitive impairment compared to people who had not had a stroke. Other data suggests that people who have survived a stroke are at double the risk of developing dementia.

Risk Factors

Many health conditions that increase your risk of cardiovascular disease also put your brain's health in jeopardy. In the following pages, we explain some of the most common risk factors for cardiovascular disease and dementia.

Obesity

According to the Centers for Disease Control and Prevention, nearly 40 percent of American adults are obese, defined as a body mass index (BMI) of 30 or higher. More than seven in 10 American adults are overweight (defined as a BMI of 25 to 29.9) or obese. Excess body weight is a key contributor to cardiovascular disease and to other heart disease and dementia risk factors, including diabetes, inflammation, and high blood pressure.

Studies have shown that overweight and obese adults are at higher risk of dementia than those who are of normal weight. Obesity has even been linked with smaller brain volume.

The relationship between weight and dementia risk is complex, however. Researchers who studied more than 1.3 million men and women reported that excess weight in earlier years is linked to a higher risk of dementia in later years. However, they also discovered that unexplained, unhealthy weight loss is linked to the onset of dementia. The researchers suggested that overweight and obesity contribute to a higher risk of dementia, but that the brain changes that occur in the very early stages of dementia may play a causative role in weight loss.

Start Early. Being overweight during later life isn't the only problem. Research also suggests that individuals who are overweight or obese in middle age are at greater risk for decreased cognitive function and dementia. In one long-running study, scientists found that being overweight or obese, measured by BMI, at age 50 was associated with earlier onset of Alzheimer's in those who developed the disease.

Extra weight also can compound the cognitive effects of other chronic health conditions. In another study, having a lower BMI was associated with better cognition when participants were first assessed. Over time, those who were both obese and suffering from conditions such as diabetes or high cholesterol were more likely to experience a faster rate of cognitive decline.

On the bright side, dropping excess pounds might help older people sharpen their mental skills. According to one study, obese people who lost weight had improved scores on tests of thinking, verbal memory, executive function, and language.

Waistline Worries. Although any excess weight is unhealthy, "belly fat" is especially dangerous, and a growing waistline can have a detrimental effect on both your heart and brain. Fat in your abdominal cavity, which is also called visceral fat, isn't the same as the subcutaneous fat that lies just beneath your skin. Visceral fat is located in the spaces between the internal organs, such as the stomach, liver, and intestines. Researchers have discovered that visceral fat cells release damaging substances that play a role in both the development of heart disease and Alzheimer's disease.

While the relationship between weight, metabolism, and diet is complicated, it remains generally true that if you consume more calories than you burn, you'll gain weight. Calories are the fuel your body, heart, and brain need to function, and they are an important nutrient in themselves. However, most Americans overdo calorie intake and don't get enough physical activity to burn off the excess calories.

In the chapters ahead, we'll show you how an eating pattern filled with nutrient-dense foods can help even the score in the trade-off between calories and other nutrients.

Hypertension

In early 2019, the American Heart Association (AHA) grabbed headlines with the news that almost half of American adults—48 percent—have heart disease, a sharp upward surge from prior years. That startling statistic needs context, however: Only 9 percent of adults have heart disease apart from hypertension, or high blood pressure.

The number of people classified as having hypertension jumped dramatically because the AHA and the American College of Cardiology changed the criteria that defines hypertension. Under the updated guidelines, hypertension is now defined as a reading of 130 millimeters of mercury (mmHg) and higher for systolic blood pressure (the top number), or a reading of 80 and higher for diastolic blood pressure (the bottom number). (The previous criteria for hypertension was a measurement of 140/90 mmHg and higher.)

Some physicians' organizations, however, continue to endorse older guidelines that set blood pressure goals at 140/90 mmHg or lower, and some also advise that people age 60 and older should be treated for hypertension only if their systolic pressure exceeds 150 mmHg.

The take-home message from these varying positions on hypertension is that you and your doctor need to discuss what

Redefining Hypertension

The American College of Cardiology and American Heart Association released new guidelines that changed the definition of high blood pressure (hypertension) to 130/80 mmHg and eliminated the category of prehypertension:

- **Normal:** Less than 120/80 mmHg
- **Elevated:** Systolic between 120–129 mmHg and diastolic less than 80 mmHg
- **Stage 1:** Systolic between 130–139 mmHg or diastolic between 80-89 mmHg
- **Stage 2:** Systolic 140 mmHg and above or diastolic 90 mmHg and above
- **Hypertensive crisis:** Systolic over 180 mmHg and/or diastolic over 120 mmHg

The American Academy of Family Physicians and American College of Physicians recommend sticking with the previous 140/90 mmHg guideline for most people. For adults age 60 and older not at high cardiovascular risk, the recommended goal is 150/90 mmHg or below.

NEW FINDING

Healthier Heart, Lower Dementia Risk

A French study of more than 6,000 older adults adds to the evidence of an association between cardiovascular health and the risk of developing dementia. The participants, average age 74, were free of cardiovascular disease and dementia at the start of the study and were followed for an average of 8.5 years.

Participants were scored using the American Heart Association's "Simple 7" factors associated with better cardiovascular health: nonsmoking, body mass index less than 25, regular physical activity, eating fish twice a week or more and fruits and vegetables at least three times a day, cholesterol below 200 mg/dL (untreated), fasting glucose below 100 mg/dL (untreated), and blood pressure below 120/80 mm Hg (untreated). The higher the number of Simple 7 factors participants had, the lower their risk of dementia.
JAMA, Aug. 21, 2018

the appropriate blood pressure target is for you, and what lifestyle measures (in addition to medication, if necessary) you should take to combat hypertension.

Effects on Body and Brain. Why is hypertension the focus of so much discussion? Because, however it's defined, high blood pressure makes the heart work harder and puts more strain on the arteries. Over time, hypertension weakens the artery walls, and it can eventually damage the muscles and valves of the heart itself, which can cause heart failure, a condition in which the heart is unable to pump an adequate amount of blood. High blood pressure also puts you at greater risk for heart attack, kidney failure, peripheral artery disease, and stroke.

Healthy BP Better for Brain

Maintaining a healthy blood pressure can help you maintain a healthy brain, according to a large study that analyzed brain health using autopsies. The study involved 1,288 people who were followed an average of eight years until their death at an average age of 88.6. A high systolic blood pressure (the top number) was associated with more brain infarcts (areas of dead tissue caused by blocked blood flow), as well as with a higher number of neurofibrillary tangles that are key markers of Alzheimer's pathology. High diastolic pressure (the bottom number) also was associated with more brain infarcts.

Neurology, Aug. 07, 2018

Tight BP Control Protects Cognition

The SPRINT study, which led some experts to lower recommendations for blood pressure targets, also provided evidence that tight blood pressure control in older adults helps reduce the risk of mild cognitive impairment (MCI), a condition in which declines in memory and thinking abilities have occurred but are not serious enough to interfere with activities of everyday life. A sub-study, SPRINT Mind, showed that meeting a systolic (top number) blood pressure target of below 120 mmHg was associated with a 19 percent lower risk of developing MCI.

The analysis included 9,361 participants ages 50 and older whose initial, untreated systolic pressure ranged from 130 to 180; all also had at least one other cardiovascular risk factor. Among participants who also underwent MRI scans, participants with tighter blood pressure control had fewer lesions in the brain's white matter. Controlling blood pressure, researchers concluded, "is not only good for the heart but also the brain."

JAMA, Jan. 28, 2019

When artery walls become weak, they are more vulnerable to damage, such as rupture and scarring. These damaged areas provide an ideal environment for plaque to accumulate, which can lead to or worsen coronary artery disease. This type of damage can affect the brain as well. In fact, high blood pressure is the leading cause of stroke and the single most important risk factor for stroke.

BP and Dementia. High blood pressure in midlife is associated with a greater risk of dementia, which may be due to mini-strokes, strokes, damage to the blood vessels, or too little blood and oxygen being delivered to the brain.

One study found that women with hypertension at an average age of 44 were 68 percent more likely to develop dementia three or four decades later than women with normal blood pressure at the same age. (In the study, the same pattern was not seen in men, although other studies have linked hypertension in men and women in their 50s to later dementia.)

Research also has shown that hypertension is associated with greater damage to the brain's white matter, which insulates and protects the neural circuits, and with disrupted activity in brain neurons—the cells that transmit information—and impaired brain function.

High Cholesterol

You probably already know that unhealthy cholesterol levels increase your risk of heart disease. Given the connections between your heart and brain, it should come as no surprise that high cholesterol also can endanger your cognitive health.

Cholesterol is a waxy substance that circulates through your blood; this is "serum" cholesterol, as opposed to dietary cholesterol, which is the cholesterol in the foods and beverages you consume. Your body, primarily your liver, makes cholesterol, which it needs for the production of cell membranes; vitamin D, hormones, and bile acids. Saturated fat in foods such as red meat, full-fat dairy foods (butter, cream, whole milk), and processed foods cause your liver to produce more cholesterol. Genetics also plays a role in how much cholesterol your body makes.

In a major shift, the current *Dietary Guidelines for Americans* dropped its previous recommendation for limiting dietary cholesterol consumption to a set amount per day. This change occurred because experts determined that dietary cholesterol is not a key contributor to the serum cholesterol in your blood vessels.

Cholesterol Effects. Excess serum cholesterol can contribute to the formation of plaque between layers of artery walls, which causes atherosclerosis and makes it harder for your heart to circulate blood. Plaque in the carotid arteries and thickening of blood vessel walls are associated with both Alzheimer's disease and vascular dementia. Other research has associated abnormal cholesterol levels in midlife with an increased risk of later dementia, including Alzheimer's.

Not all serum cholesterol is harmful. The low-density lipoprotein (LDL) form of cholesterol is the type associated with arterial plaque buildup. Conversely, beneficial high-density lipoprotein (HDL) cholesterol carries LDL cholesterol away from the arteries and back to the liver, where it is broken down into waste products and eliminated from the body. HDL cholesterol also might help preserve memory by reducing the formation of beta-amyloid, a substance that clusters to form plaques in the brains of people with Alzheimer's disease.

Diabetes and Insulin Resistance

Diabetes is a risk factor for heart disease, and research suggests it's also bad for the brain. A 2018 study reported that both prediabetes and diabetes, which are characterized by elevated blood glucose levels, are tied to a faster rate of cognitive decline (problems with memory, concentration, making and executing decisions, and difficulty learning new things) than normal blood glucose levels. The study showed a linear association between HbA1c status—a test that shows what average glucose levels have been during the three months preceding the test—and long-term cognitive decline: As blood glucose levels rose, so did the risk of decline.

In another study, researchers compared the results of MRI brain scans and cognitive tests conducted on type 2 diabetes patients along with control subjects who did not have diabetes. Participants with diabetes had more white-matter abnormalities in the brain than the control group, and they scored lower on tests of memory and reaction times.

How Diabetes Develops. Type 2 diabetes, which usually develops in adulthood, typically starts with a condition called insulin resistance. When you consume carbohydrates, your digestive system breaks down their component sugars and starches into a simple sugar called glucose. Insulin, a hormone produced by the pancreas, acts like a "key" to unlock the body's cells so glucose can pass from the blood into the cells and be used as energy or stored as fat. Insulin resistance occurs when the cell receptors that respond to insulin no longer work as well—no matter how much insulin the pancreas produces, glucose can't exit from the bloodstream, and levels go up.

Maintaining a healthy weight and being physically active are the most effective ways to prevent insulin resistance. Most people who are overweight are also insulin resistant, although a small number of lean people also develop insulin resistance, likely for genetic reasons.

When blood glucose levels remain high over time, the pancreas cannot produce enough insulin to handle the excess glucose; consequently, blood glucose levels remain elevated, and a patient may be diagnosed with prediabetes. Finally, the condition may progress to type 2 diabetes.

What Diabetes Does. High blood glucose prevents the blood vessels from opening (dilating) wide enough to let blood flow through easily. This contributes to increased plaque buildup, heart disease, and impaired blood flow to the brain, as well as to all other organs and tissues.

Insulin resistance may in turn lead to high blood pressure. Excess insulin may cause the kidneys to retain more sodium, which increases the fluid volume in the arteries, resulting in elevated blood pressure.

Chronically high blood glucose levels have been linked with an increased risk of dementia. One group of researchers reported that study participants with very high blood glucose levels were at 23 percent greater risk of dementia than those with lower levels. Even study

Blood Glucose by the Numbers

Doctors may check your fasting blood glucose (FBG) or glycated hemoglobin (HbA1c) level to determine whether you have diabetes or prediabetes.

FBG RESULT	CONDITION
70–99 mg/dL	Normal
100–125 mg/dL	Prediabetes
126 mg/dL or higher	Diabetes

HBA1C RESULT	CONDITION
Below 5.7%	Normal
5.7% to 6.4%	Prediabetes
6.5% or higher	Diabetes

Eat Right for a Bigger Brain

Can a healthy diet actually result in a bigger brain? That's the suggestion of a long-running Dutch study that compared adherence to dietary guidelines with MRI brain scans over a 10-year span. The study looked at 4,231 participants in the Rotterdam Study, average age 66 at the beginning of the study. A healthy diet was measured by how closely participants adhered to official Dutch recommendations on consumption of vegetables, fruit, whole grains, legumes, nuts, dairy, fish, tea, unsaturated fats and oils, red and processed meat, sugary beverages, alcohol, and salt. After adjusting for other risk factors, a healthier diet was linked to larger total brain volume, gray matter volume, white matter volume, and hippocampal volume.

The healthy diet, researchers noted, resembles the Mediterranean diet. They added, "The scientific literature thus far indicates that a balanced diet pattern rich in healthy carbs and fiber, with low-to-moderate fat content, is supportive of brain aging. There is no evidence for the opposite, which provides a strong argument in favor of recommending a Mediterranean-style diet for brain aging and dementia prevention."

Neurology, May 16, 2018

participants with elevated blood glucose levels that were not high enough for a diagnosis of diabetes were 20 percent more likely to develop dementia than those with normal blood glucose levels. Excess glucose might damage brain function by altering components of neurons, increasing oxidative stress, and producing inflammation.

Another possible factor is an enzyme involved in regulating insulin. The enzyme that breaks down insulin also works to break down beta-amyloid, a compound that accumulates in the brains of people with Alzheimer's disease. Scientists speculate that when the enzyme is attacking excess insulin, beta-amyloid may be left to build up in damaging plaques in the brain.

Improving Heart-Brain Health

It's never too soon to start taking better care of your heart and brain, even if you're not yet a "senior citizen" and the possibilities of heart disease and dementia seem years away. Consider one study of cardiovascular risk factors and the amyloid deposits in the brain associated with Alzheimer's disease: Researchers analyzed data on initially healthy participants with a mean age of 52 years in a long-running study of more than two decades. At the study's end, brain scans showed that people who had risk factors for cardiovascular disease at the study's outset were more likely to have elevated amyloid levels more than 20 years later. Risk factors included smoking, hypertension, diabetes, unhealthy cholesterol levels, and obesity.

On the other hand, even if you're older, it's not too late to make changes now that can benefit your heart and brain in the years ahead. For example, one study assessed whether lifestyle changes had an effect on the cognitive function of adults ages 60 to 77. Half of the study participants were randomly assigned to an intervention including dietary changes, exercise, cognitive training, and vascular risk monitoring, while the other half, the control group, was merely given general health advice. After two years, the intervention group had a 25 percent greater improvement in total scores of cognitive function than the control group.

Another study found that people who engaged in unhealthy behaviors (smoking, low fruit and vegetable consumption, low amount of physical activity, and high alcohol consumption) were nearly three times more likely to suffer impairments in thinking and twice as likely to have memory problems as those with the fewest bad habits. Compared to those with zero unhealthy behaviors, participants with three or four unhealthy behaviors were 84 percent more likely to have poor cognitive function 17 years later.

It's clear that the choices you make today—whatever your age—can affect your future risk of cardiovascular disease and cognitive decline. Those smart choices start with how you feed your heart and brain—as we'll see in the next chapter.

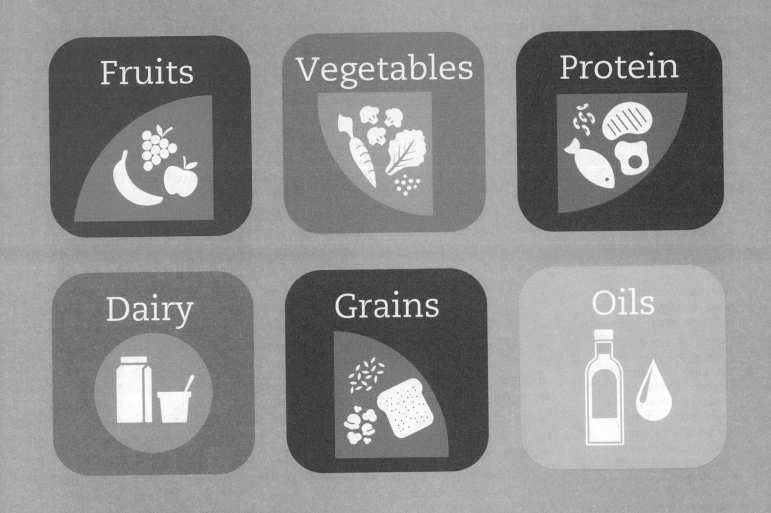

2 Patterns for Protection

Your total dietary pattern has a significant impact on your heart and brain health.

We know more about what makes up a heart-healthy dietary pattern than we do about "brain food," although research on nutrition and cognition is making important progress.

The word "pattern" deserves special attention. It's important to focus on your overall eating pattern instead of thinking solely in terms of individual foods or nutrients. A diet that helps protect your heart and brain involves more than just eating an extra serving of broccoli and occasionally choosing grilled chicken instead of a cheeseburger. The most recent *Dietary Guidelines for Americans* (DGA) explains: "An eating pattern is more than the sum of its parts; it represents the totality of what individuals habitually eat and drink, and these dietary components act synergistically in relation to health. As a result, the eating pattern may be more predictive of overall health status and disease risk than individual foods or nutrients."

Cardiovascular disease is high on the list of chronic diseases that a healthy dietary pattern can help prevent—and we've already seen how a healthy heart and vascular system can help protect your brain.

A Heart-Healthy Pattern

What does a dietary pattern that's healthy for your heart look like? According to the Dietary Guidelines Advisory Committee report, a "healthy dietary

Med-Style Diet Linked with Better Brain Function

Researchers have found that following a Mediterranean-style diet may improve cognitive function in people with diabetes. In the study, the participants' diets were scored according to how similar they were to a Mediterranean-style diet, a DASH diet, and two healthy eating indices, and they were given several cognitive tests. Two years later, the participants were again given the cognitive tests.

The participants who had diabetes and glycemic levels that were stable or improved and followed a Mediterranean-style diet scored better on cognitive tests that measured executive and memory function as well as global cognition. However, those who had diabetes and poor or declined glycemic control and followed a Mediterranean-style diet did not have improved scores on cognitive tests. Study participants who did not have diabetes scored higher on memory tests if their diets were similar to any of the four healthy dietary patterns scored in the study.

Diabetes Care, May 2019

pattern is higher in vegetables, fruits, whole grains, low- or nonfat dairy, seafood, legumes, and nuts, moderate in alcohol (among adults), lower in red and processed meats, and low in sugar-sweetened foods and drinks and refined grains."

If you think a heart-healthy dietary pattern includes a strict limit on fat, think again. Based on updates in the science of how different fats affect health, the DGA overturned the previous 30 years of recommendations regarding dietary fat. In the last update, the DGA did not set a recommended limit on total fat consumption; instead, the focus shifted to the type of fat in your diet.

The DGA still advises limiting intake of saturated fat, found in foods such as red and processed meats, butter, and whole-fat dairy foods. (The recommendation about limiting dairy fat is now controversial, however, with some research showing little reason to avoid whole-fat dairy.)

Nutrition experts emphasize choosing more foods that contain unsaturated fat, such as vegetable oils, nuts, seeds, avocados, and fish rich in omega-3 fats. This change is in keeping with dietary patterns that have been linked with lower risks of chronic disease, such as a Mediterranean-style diet, which contains healthy amounts of unsaturated fat but is low in saturated fat.

"Brain Food"

Evidence is mounting for the idea that what you eat also can help protect your brain. Fewer studies have investigated the connection between diet and brain function than between diet and heart health, but the existing research does suggest that certain dietary patterns can make a difference in your brain's ability to store, access, and retrieve information, formulate and execute plans, and make decisions.

One study, for example, found that diets high in anti-inflammatory foods were linked with a lower risk of cognitive decline and impairment. Diets that were higher in phytonutrient-rich fruits and vegetables, whole grains, and fiber were anti-inflammatory, while diets that were higher in saturated and trans fats were pro-inflammatory.

Going Mediterranean

In the annual diet rankings published by the *U.S. News and World Report*, the Mediterranean diet took top honors for the best overall diet as well as the best diet for healthy eating, and the DGA specifically recommends this dietary pattern. Many studies have found associations between a Mediterranean-style dietary pattern and better cardiovascular health.

While you've probably heard of the "Mediterranean diet," you might not know what this term really means—and the name can be a bit confusing if you associate "Mediterranean" food with the fare offered at modern Italian or Greek eateries. Many American restaurants have "Westernized" traditional Mediterranean cuisine, resulting in dishes that are high in saturated fat and calories (think pizza with pepperoni and extra cheese or fettuccine Alfredo) and fewer vegetables, whole grains, and legumes.

When you think of a Mediterranean-style diet, think instead of the traditional fare consumed by the people of the Mediterranean region in countries such as Crete, Greece, and southern Italy around 1960. At that time, the rates of chronic disease in these Mediterranean countries were among the lowest in the world, and adult life expectancy was among the highest. The dietary pattern, which consisted mainly of fruits and vegetables, beans and nuts, healthy grains, fish, olive oil, small amounts of dairy, and red wine, proved to be much more likely to lead to lifelong good health than dietary patterns that contain more meat and processed foods and fewer fruits and vegetables.

Unlike fad diets that promise a quick fix but can't be sustained over time, the Mediterranean-style diet isn't difficult to stick to—it's easy to integrate into an overall healthy lifestyle that can be maintained for the rest of your life.

A traditional Mediterranean-style diet is filled with a variety of delicious, satisfying foods, including olive oil, nuts, and other plant foods that are rich in healthy, unsaturated fat. Moderate alcohol intake—especially of red wine—is allowed. This dietary pattern also is notable for what it doesn't include: highly processed foods.

What the Science Says

Numerous studies have reported that adhering to a Mediterranean-style diet is associated with a reduced risk of stroke and heart attack, lower LDL ("bad") cholesterol levels, and less likelihood of obesity. Research also has linked brain benefits with following a Mediterranean-style eating pattern.

In one study, participants assigned to follow a Mediterranean-style diet scored better in tests of global cognition, executive function, and memory than a control group who was advised only to reduce fat intake. Another study reported that participants who included more fish and plant foods in their diets while eating less red meat and dairy were less likely to develop cognitive impairment.

Even countries in which the traditional eating patterns are very different from those of Mediterranean countries

NEW FINDING

Stroke Risk Lower on Mediterranean Diet

Eating like a Mediterranean may reduce the risk of stroke, especially for women. In a UK study of more than 23,000 adults, women over 40 who most closely adhered to a Mediterranean diet were 22 percent less likely to suffer a stroke over 17 years of follow-up. Men who followed the diet were at 6 percent lower risk; overall, the diet was associated with a 17 percent risk reduction.

"Our study tells us there are differences between men and women and risk of stroke with the Mediterranean-style diet," researchers commented. "We do not know yet why this is, but the components of the diet may influence men differently than women." They added that the synergistic ways in which nutrients worked together seemed to be more important than specific components of the diet.

Stroke, Sept. 20, 2018

Mediterranean Diet Pyramid

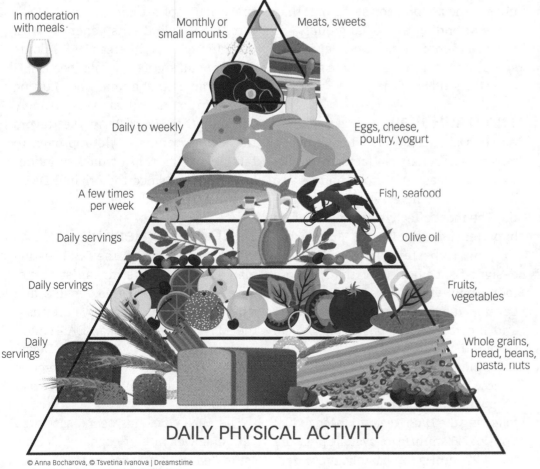

In moderation with meals

Monthly or small amounts — Meats, sweets

Daily to weekly — Eggs, cheese, poultry, yogurt

A few times per week — Fish, seafood

Daily servings — Olive oil

Daily servings — Fruits, vegetables

Daily servings — Whole grains, bread, beans, pasta, nuts

DAILY PHYSICAL ACTIVITY

© Anna Bocharova, © Tsvetina Ivanova | Dreamstime

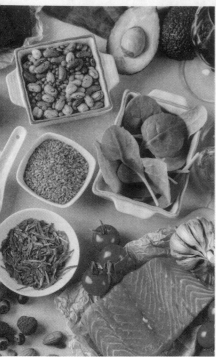

© Aamulya | Dreamstime

A Mediterranean-style diet consists mainly of whole grains, fruits, vegetables, nuts, fish, and beans. Olive oil is the primary source of fat, and red wine can be enjoyed in moderation.

report brain benefits of adopting a Mediterranean-style diet. In a Scottish study of older adults, those who ate the most fruits, vegetables, olive oil, and other Mediterranean-style fare and the least fried food, red meat, and cheese had about half the expected rate of brain shrinkage as participants who ate traditional Scottish fare.

Another clinical trial suggests that the Mediterranean-style diet also might help protect your mental health. Researchers randomly assigned more than 100 adults with depression to receive either Mediterranean foods and fish oil supplements and take a Mediterranean cooking class every other week, or to attend social groups every other week. After three months, the Mediterranean-diet group was eating more vegetables, fruit, nuts, whole grains, and legumes, fewer unhealthy snacks, and less red meat.

Participants in the Mediterranean diet group experienced greater reductions in their depression symptoms than those attending the social groups. The improvements in diet and depressive symptoms held steady three months after the study ended.

The DASH Plan

As we saw in the previous chapter, hypertension is a primary risk factor for cardiovascular disease and stroke, and it's also linked with an increased risk of dementia. The most effective diet for reducing hypertension—the Dietary Approaches to Stop Hypertension (DASH)—was designed specifically for that purpose more than two decades ago. DASH was developed by the National Heart, Lung and Blood Institute based on clinical studies that tested the effects of sodium and other nutrients on blood pressure.

How much can your blood pressure drop with the DASH diet? In one study, following the DASH diet produced reductions of 7.62 mmHg for systolic pressure and 4.22 mmHg for diastolic pressure.

Even if you don't have high blood pressure, DASH is a healthy way to eat. In the decades since DASH was developed, numerous studies have linked the diet with a host of health benefits, including reduced risks of coronary heart disease, stroke, and heart failure. And the DASH diet was ranked second in the 2019 *U.S. News and World Report* rankings of healthy diets (the Mediterranean-style diet was ranked first).

DASH Ingredients

The DASH diet is high in fruits, vegetables, and low-fat dairy. It emphasizes whole grains, fish, poultry, and nuts and limits red meats, added sugars, and sodium. Overall, the plan is rich in phytonutrients, potassium, magnesium, calcium, and fiber. For a complete guide to the DASH diet, see https://tinyurl.com/yc2n5lfd.

There are many similarities between DASH and a Mediterranean-style diet, but there is one important difference: the amount of fat consumed. A Mediterranean-style diet is generous with unsaturated fats, whereas DASH limits fats from all sources (remember, DASH was formulated at a time when cutting consumption of all fat was strongly advised). Our Heart-Brain Diet favors the Mediterranean-style approach to fats, in recognition of dietary guidelines updated since the original DASH research was conducted.

MIND Melds Healthy Diets

We've seen that both the DASH eating plan and the Mediterranean-style diet have been linked to brain benefits, and a hybrid of these two dietary patterns—the "MIND" (Mediterranean-DASH Intervention for Neurodegenerative Delay) diet—may be even better at protecting memory and thinking than either diet on its own.

The MIND diet has been associated with a slower rate of cognitive decline estimated to be equivalent to 7.5 years of younger mental age. These results were based on data from participants in the Rush Memory and Aging Project, ages 58 to 98, who were initially free of Alzheimer's disease. Other studies have found a lower incidence of Alzheimer's disease in people who closely adhered to the MIND diet.

Stroke and Dementia Risk

The MIND diet also might help stroke survivors ward off cognitive decline, according to 2018 research. In general, people who have had a stroke are twice as likely to develop dementia as the general population, but researchers discovered that stroke survivors whose diets most closely resembled the MIND diet had substantially slower rates of cognitive decline than those whose diets were least similar to the MIND diet.

Stroke survivors who scored high on the Mediterranean and DASH diets, however, did not have significant slowing in their cognitive decline. Researchers commented, "The Mediterranean and DASH diets have been shown to be protective against coronary artery disease and stroke, but it seems the nutrients emphasized in the MIND diet may be better suited to overall brain health and preserving cognition." These include folate, vitamin E, omega-3 fatty acids, carotenoids, and flavonoids.

Making a MIND Diet

Why might the MIND diet be protective?

"Inflammation and oxidative stress play a large role in the development and progression of Alzheimer's disease," says Tammy Scott, PhD, a scientist at Tufts' HNRCA Neuroscience and Aging Laboratory and consulting editor for this report. "The MIND diet particularly emphasizes foods such as green leafy vegetables, berries, and olive oil that are rich in antioxidants and anti-inflammatory agents that may help to protect against dementia and cognitive decline."

Key ingredients in the MIND diet include:

- **Green leafy vegetables:** at least six servings per week
- **Other vegetables:** at least one serving per day
- **Berries:** at least two servings per week
- **Nuts:** at least five servings per week
- **Olive oil** as the primary cooking oil
- **Whole grains:** at least three servings per day
- **Fish (not fried):** at least once per week
- **Beans:** more than three meals per week
- **Chicken or turkey (not fried):** at least two meals per week
- **Wine:** one glass per day (optional)

Researchers noted that it's as important to limit unhealthy foods as it is to eat healthy foods. The MIND diet recommends having less than one serving a week of red meat, cheese, fried or fast food, and pastries and sweets, and less than one tablespoon of butter a day.

Skip the Fads

The DASH, Mediterranean-style, and MIND diets are hardly the only plans promising heart and brain benefits. Plenty of fad diets claim to quickly and easily boost your heart health, melt off extra pounds, and even boost your memory. Most have some nuggets of good advice, but many go to extremes, and some may have potentially dangerous side effects. Do these diets have anything to offer for a healthy heart and brain?

Low-Carb Craze

Average Americans didn't give "carbs" much thought until the Atkins "diet revolution." Proponents of low-carbohydrate diets claim that eating fewer carbs forces your body to burn stored fat for energy. When you digest carbs, your body converts them to sugar in the form of glucose that goes into your bloodstream. Rising blood glucose levels prompt your body to produce more insulin, which transports the glucose from

NEW FINDING

MIND Diet May Help Stroke Survivors

The MIND diet, a hybrid of the DASH and Mediterranean diets that emphasizes brain-healthy foods, has been shown to slow cognitive decline. A new observational study tested whether a similar benefit might be seen in stroke survivors; people who have suffered a stroke and survived are twice as likely to develop dementia as the general population.

The study followed 108 stroke survivors for almost five years. The researchers determined how closely the survivors adhered to the MIND diet and analyzed results from a battery of 19 cognitive tests. Participants who scored highest for MIND diet adherence had substantially slower rates of cognitive decline than those who scored lowest. The apparent effect of the diet remained strong even after taking into account participants' level of education and their degree of participation in cognitive and physical activities. Similar benefits were not associated with adherence to either the Mediterranean or DASH diets, however.

Neurology, April 24, 2018

your blood into your cells for energy. When you restrict carb consumption, you have less glucose in your blood, so your body must use stored fat for energy instead.

But it's important to consider the valuable nutrients found in many carbohydrate-containing foods before taking them off the menu. Going "low-carb" means restricting healthy whole grains, fruits, vegetables, legumes, milk, and yogurt. Some research suggests that eating too few carbohydrates might deny your brain the nutrients it needs to think clearly, so decreasing carbs also may decrease cognitive performance.

Just as with fat, the current thinking on carbs emphasizes the type of carbs you eat, rather than the amount. It is true that research suggests foods high in refined carbohydrates, such as white flour and added sugar, contribute to weight gain and diabetes risk. Since both of these conditions are unhealthy for your heart and brain, it's wise to watch out for these types of carbs. Our Heart-Brain Diet emphasizes healthy, unprocessed carbohydrates that are packed with essential nutrients.

What About "Keto"? The latest weight-loss craze is the "ketogenic" or "keto" diet, which is similar to the extremely low-carbohydrate diet popularized by Atkins in the 1970s and again by the South Beach diet in the early 2000s. By sharply restricting carbohydrates, the keto diet forces the body to get energy from fat, which results in a release of ketones into the bloodstream. Like the Atkins diet, a keto diet is rich in proteins and fats and may be lacking in nutritious fruits, vegetables, and whole grains. The keto diet is very restrictive and it often causes fatigue, so most people don't follow it for long. It also can be dangerous for people with kidney disease, and some doctors caution that strict adherence to a keto diet for longer than a few weeks can contribute to loss of muscle mass and heart damage.

Following the keto diet usually results in rapid weight loss, but many people regain some or all of the weight they lost once they stop the diet. Interestingly, a keto diet helps ease epilepsy symptoms in some children, but the mechanism of this effect in unclear, and speculation that the diet might have brain benefits for adults has not been supported by human studies.

Forget Low-Fat Eating

We've already mentioned the change in thinking about fats: Low-fat diets are out, and healthy fats are in. The low-fat, highly processed foods made by food manufacturers in the 1980s usually contained increased sugar, salt, and/or refined carbs to compensate for the reduction in fat. Eating these low-fat junk foods didn't improve people's diets; instead, they contributed to what has become an obesity epidemic.

It's true that following a low-fat diet might mean consuming fewer calories, since fats are a concentrated form of calories—nine calories per gram, compared to four calories per gram of protein or carbohydrate. If you replace those fats with refined carbohydrates, however, you'll quickly make up for any initial calorie reduction. Foods that contain fat provide a feeling of satiety and long-lasting fullness that makes it easier to control your appetite—an effect that you won't get from refined carbs.

Our heart-brain diet emphasizes healthy, mono- and polyunsaturated fats from a variety of foods including nuts, vegetable oils, seeds, avocados, and cold-water fatty fish.

Low-Carb Versus Low-Fat. Studies have found that low-carb and low-fat diets work equally well for weight loss, at least in the short term. Experts advise that any diet you find easy to stick to—which is typically true of those with a simple "eat less of this" mantra—can be effective. Neither low-carb nor low-fat eating is a nutritious prescription for lifelong health, however.

While it's true that any diet plan that is too permissive won't help you control your weight or protect your heart and brain, it's also true that any diet that forces you to deny yourself all of the foods you love is likely to be short-lived. The heart-brain diet incorporates both moderation and balance, so it is both effective and sustainable; it even includes desserts.

Eating Like a Caveman

Another recent fad is the "Paleo" diet, which claims to emulate the "natural" diet of humans who lived in the Paleolithic period, commonly called the "Stone Age." Anthropologists have pointed out, however, that the actual diets of early humans were varied and opportunistic—in other words, they ate what they could find. If early humans were less prone to "diseases of affluence" such as heart disease, it's likely because they died too young to develop such conditions. Also, some foods endorsed by Paleo promoters were not actually available to our Paleolithic forebears.

The Paleo diet emphasizes grass-fed meats, fish and seafood, fresh fruits and vegetables, eggs, nuts and seeds, and unrefined oils from nuts, seeds, olives, avocados, and coconuts. Some of these foods are healthy, but in practice, the Paleo diet gives followers an excuse to eat a lot of meat. The danger of eating large amounts of meat is the excessive saturated fat content—the leading dietary cause of unhealthy LDL cholesterol levels.

Paleo followers avoid cereal grains, legumes, most dairy products, refined vegetable oils, processed foods, sugar and other commercial sweeteners, and salt. It's smart to cut down on sugar, salt, and processed foods, but whole grains, legumes, and dairy foods are important sources of nutrients. In particular, grains and legumes are good sources of slowly digested carbohydrates that give your body the steady supply of energy it requires.

As for sugars, there's little evidence that the Paleo approach of choosing "natural" sweeteners, such as agave nectar, date sugar, honey, or maple syrup, rather than granulated sugar or other commercial sweeteners, has health benefits. All of these sweeteners contain roughly the same amount of calories and affect the body similarly.

Another issue is that most Paleo diets don't set any limits for calories. In our calorie-rich modern world, failing to limit calories in any dietary regimen can lead to weight gain and obesity.

The bottom line is that the Paleo diet doesn't accurately reflect what our cave-dwelling ancestors consumed, and it doesn't contain the balance of carbs, proteins, and fats we need to keep the hearts and brains in our 21st-century bodies healthy. And the Paleo diet has not been endorsed by the American Diabetes Association, the American Heart Association, or any other large, reputable health organizations.

Vegetarian Options

Although vegetarian and vegan diets also have been growing in popularity, this does not make them "fad diets." The benefits of plant-based dietary patterns have been solidly backed by science, and the latest dietary guidelines include a vegetarian diet as an example of a healthy dietary pattern. Eating vegan or vegetarian has been associated with lower risks of obesity, cardiovascular disease, and type 2 diabetes. Such diets tend to be lower in saturated fat than traditional Western diets, and they tend to provide more fiber, phytonutrients, and antioxidants.

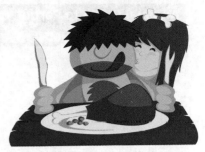

© Arleevector | Dreamstime

The Paleo diet claims to be based on what our cave-dwelling ancestors ate, but they were hunter-gatherers, and they didn't all share a common diet. Their location and environment determined whether their diet was high in meat, fish, plants, or other foods.

A Visual Guide to Portion Sizes

FOOD	SERVING	WHAT IT LOOKS LIKE
Cereal	1 cup	Baseball
Salad greens	1 cup	Fist
Cooked rice or pasta	½ cup	Half of a baseball
Ice cream	½ cup	Half of a baseball
Peanut butter	2 Tbsp	Ping pong ball
Meat, poultry	3 ounces	Deck of cards
Fish	3 ounces	Checkbook
Cheese	1½ ounces	4 dice

Switching to a vegetarian diet doesn't guarantee weight loss or heart-brain health, however. You still need to make smart food choices. Replacing meat with highly processed foods, such as white pasta and bread, snack chips, protein bars, and sweets, may cause you to gain weight, and it won't lead to any health benefits.

Aim to eat whole foods as often as possible, including plenty of vegetables, fruits, legumes, and whole grains, and limit processed foods that contain sodium, added sugar, saturated fat, and refined grains, such as white flour. Vegetarians and vegans also need to ensure that they're getting enough of certain essential nutrients, including iron, vitamin B_{12}, vitamin D, calcium, zinc, and omega-3 fatty acids, since animal foods are the primary sources of these nutrients. Some people choose a lacto-ovo-vegetarian diet, which includes eggs, milk, and milk products; this dietary pattern lessens your chances of having a calcium deficiency.

Some research has shown that a pescatarian diet, which includes fish along with an abundance of plant foods, may be even healthier than strict vegetarian eating. Such a plan also may be easier to stick to for people used to eating animal protein. If you just can't give up burgers and steaks, make sure they're the exception rather than the rule.

Practice Portion Control

Finding a dietary pattern that works for you is only part of eating healthy for your heart and brain. Even good-for-you foods can be consumed in excess, so you need to practice portion control. It's not difficult to understand why most Americans eat too much: Beverages and fries at fast-food joints have been "super-sized," and meals at many restaurants easily can feed two or three people. And many people don't stop to consider if they are full; they just keep on eating until the food is gone. Add to this the fact that food is easily accessible for most Americans, and it's clear why so many Americans are overweight or obese.

Here are a few tips to help you keep portions in perspective:

▶ **Read food labels when grocery shopping.** When a package says it contains more than one serving, measure out one serving into a separate dish. Not all serving sizes listed on Nutrition Facts labels reflect how much most people serve themselves, so don't be fooled.

▶ **Practice "mindful eating."** Take time to focus on and enjoy the tastes, textures, and aromas of your food. Avoid eating in front of the TV or computer or while using your tablet or smartphone.

▶ **Serve food on smaller plates.** Instead of using a dinner plate, substitute a luncheon plate or a salad plate.

▶ **When eating at home,** put reasonable portions of food on your plate and keep the rest of the food in the kitchen. Then, if you want to eat more, you'll have to make a conscious decision to go get it. (What's a "reasonable" portion? See our guide to portion sizes on this page.)

▶ **When eating out,** keep in mind that restaurant portion sizes are often at least double, and sometimes triple, the amount you should be eating. As soon as your meal arrives, divide it in half and box up one half, or share it with a dining companion.

Staying Hydrated

In addition to nutritious food, your heart and brain need plenty of fluids to function properly. You lose water every day through your breath, sweat, and urine, and you need to replenish what you lose. The Institute of Medicine says that, in general, women may need 91 ounces (about 11 cups) of water daily, and men may need 125 ounces (about 15½ cups) of water daily. That's even more than the eight glasses of water per day you may have heard you need. Your diet contains many sources of water, however, including coffee, tea, and milk, along with fruits and vegetables, and even grains, poultry, and seafood, which all contribute to your daily fluid needs.

Most people can let thirst be their guide to adequate hydration without counting glasses of water. However, as you get older, you may need to pay closer attention to ensure you're getting enough fluids, because your sense of thirst may decline with age. Be alert for signs that it's time for a drink—urinating infrequently, less urine output than usual, dark-yellow or brown urine, and/or a dry mouth.

Choose calorie-free beverages, such as water and unsweetened tea and coffee, to limit your intake of added sugar and empty calories. Low-fat and skim milk are other nutrient-dense choices with a moderate calorie count.

Questions on Diet Drinks

One way people cut down on calories in their beverages is by switching to artificially sweetened sodas. According to the U.S. Food and Drug Administration, "Food safety experts generally agree there is no convincing evidence of a cause-and-effect relationship between these sweeteners and negative health effects in humans." Questions have been raised, however, about whether non-caloric sweeteners somehow might contribute to weight gain, and some studies have linked diet sodas and drinks to serious health problems.

One study did find that some people who drank diet soda daily were almost three times as likely to suffer a stroke and develop dementia as those who consumed diet soda weekly or less often. However, the media's report of this study may have caused undue alarm.

Tufts expert Tammy Scott, PhD, cautions, "The results of this study show no dose response; that is, the people who drank two to six artificially sweetened drinks per day were not more likely to have a stroke than those who had only one a day. More importantly, while those who drank one a day were three times more likely to develop dementia, those drinking two to six per day did not have an increased risk over those who drank zero artificially sweetened drinks. Another concern is that when the investigators controlled for diabetes and obesity, the association between artificially sweetened drinks and stroke/dementia was reduced." This finding could mean that people who have diabetes or are obese may be more likely to drink artificially sweetened beverages rather than sugar-sweetened ones, and it's the diabetes and obesity rather than the beverages that raise the risk for stroke and dementia.

While the current evidence falls short of making the case to avoid all artificially sweetened beverages, such concerns do support advice to make water your first choice for staying hydrated.

Fluids in Fruits and Veggies

When calculating your daily fluid intake, don't forget about the water found naturally in foods. Many fruits and vegetables are composed of more than 90 percent water. Examples include:

- Apples
- Bell peppers
- Broccoli
- Cabbage
- Cantaloupe
- Carrots
- Cauliflower
- Cucumbers
- Eggplant
- Grapefruit
- Grapes
- Lettuce
- Oranges
- Pears
- Pineapple
- Raspberries
- Spinach
- Strawberries
- Tomatoes
- Watermelon

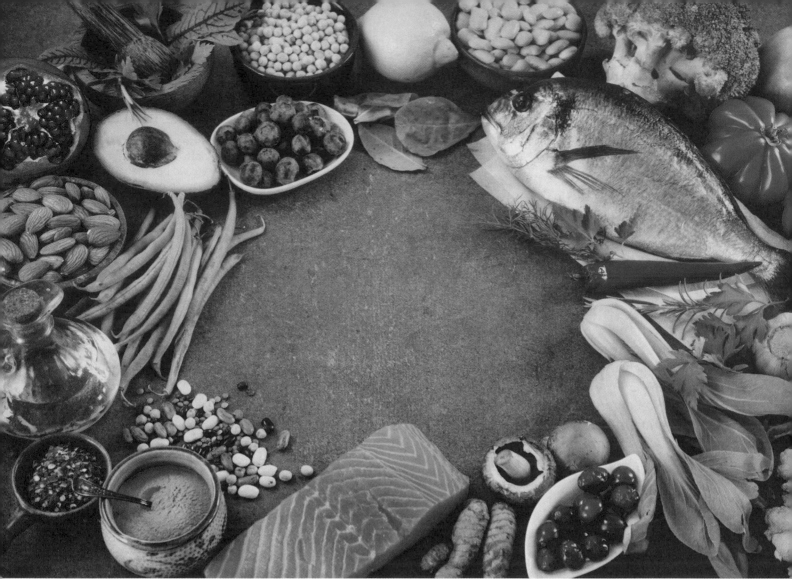

© Alexander Raths | Dreamstime

Fill your healthy eating pattern with a wide variety of nutrient-dense foods.

3 Healthy Choices

Despite their differences and colorful names, the recommended diet plans we looked at in the previous chapter have many similarities. All emphasize getting more nutrients from plants than most Americans currently do, and most call for more seafood than many Americans eat.

These heart-brain healthy choices are all "nutrient dense" rather than "energy-dense." In terms of nutrition, "energy" equals calories, so foods that are energy-dense contain a lot of calories for the amount of food. For example, the popular snack food Twinkies has 250 calories in two cakes that weigh 77 grams. One-half cup of chopped broccoli weighing 78 grams provides 27 calories and, of

course, the broccoli's nutrient content is much higher than the Twinkies, despite its extremely low calorie load.

In general, nutrient-dense foods include vegetables, fruits, whole grains, seafood, eggs, beans and peas, nuts and seeds, dairy products, and lean meats and poultry. Most processed foods are not nutrient-dense, since they have been "diluted" by the addition of calories from animal fats, sugars, sodium, and/or refined grains.

Even healthy foods contain calories, and if you eat too many calories, you will gain weight and increase your risk of cardiovascular disease and cognitive decline. That's why nutrition experts advise choosing nutrient-dense foods, which deliver many important vitamins, minerals, and other nutrients, rather than energy-dense choices that are packed with calories and little else.

Smart Trade-Offs

This concept of nutrient density can be helpful when you're making everyday food choices. Consider that a cup of peaches and five ounces of non-diet cola each contains about 60 calories. The peach provides fiber, vitamins A and C, potassium, and phytonutrients called carotenoids—it's a nutrient-dense food. Conversely, the cola is energy-dense (high in calories) because of its high sugar content, but it provides no healthy nutrients. (Foods high in calories and low in nutrients also may be called "empty-calorie" foods.) Clearly, the healthier choice is the peach.

Even among healthy whole foods, some choices are more nutrient-dense than others. For example, substituting romaine or red leaf lettuce in place of iceberg lettuce can boost your nutrient intake. Salmon contains more omega-3 fatty acids than tilapia, one of America's most popular farmed fish. (However, tilapia still can be a smart choice, especially if you're eating it instead of a protein higher in calories and saturated fat, such as a ribeye steak.)

Favor Fruits and Veggies

You already know that fruits and vegetables are good for you, and you may have heard that you should aim for five servings each day. However, results from an analysis of almost 100 studies suggest that "five a day" is just a good start—and eating 10 daily servings of produce is more beneficial. The analysis revealed that consuming five servings of fruits and vegetables daily was associated with a 14 percent lower risk of heart disease, compared to consuming no servings—but eating 10 servings a day was associated with a 24 percent

lower risk. (A serving was one-half cup cooked vegetables or a small piece of fruit.) Produce most strongly linked to lower cardiovascular risk included leafy greens, cruciferous vegetables (such as broccoli and cabbage), citrus fruits, apples, and pears.

Another study found that people who consumed the most fruits and vegetables (seven or more daily servings) were 31 percent less likely to die of cardiovascular disease than people who consumed less than one daily serving.

Even though more is better, some produce is better than none: A Chinese study found that eating about 3.5 ounces of fruit daily was associated with a 30 percent lower risk of death from cardiovascular causes. That amount is roughly equivalent to one cup of sliced fruit, such as apples or peaches, 20 grapes, a little less than a full cup of berries, or one small, whole fruit, such as an orange or a pear.

Research on Specific Produce

Fruits and vegetables are smart, nutrient-dense choices because they are relatively low in calories and free of saturated fat, and they contain vitamins, minerals, fiber, and phytonutrients. You can choose whichever fruits and vegetables you like most, though it's a good idea to eat a wide variety.

Some research has focused on the heart and brain benefits of specific types of fruits and vegetables. For example:

▶ **Apples** may help protect against stroke. In one study, adding just one apple a day to a healthy diet reduced blood levels of LDL cholesterol by about 40 percent.

▶ **Avocados** have been associated with improved cholesterol levels, and they are good sources of healthy unsaturated fats.

▶ **Beans and other legumes,** collectively known as "pulses," may benefit your heart and brain by lowering your LDL

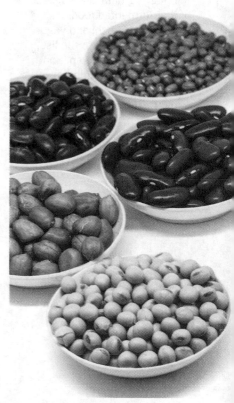

© Nattawat Kaewjirasit | Dreamstime

Pulses—beans, peas, and lentils—may help lower your LDL cholesterol.

Hype vs. Hope in Heart-Health Foods

What should physicians tell their patients about foods hyped for heart health? A review for the American College of Cardiology says some of these trendy foods actually do have cardiovascular benefits. Those that the experts concluded might be helpful to heart health were:

- Mushrooms
- Legumes
- Coffee in moderation
- Tea
- Modest alcohol intake for drinkers
- Vitamin B$_{12}$ supplements, albeit "not in excess, and when dietary deficiencies are present."
- Omega-3 fatty acids from plant or marine sources.

Emerging data also suggest that fermented foods, including kimchi and yogurt, could be added to the list. The experts were split on dairy products, citing mixed findings and controversies over full-fat dairy's health effects.

Journal of the American College of Cardiology, July 2018

level. Pulses include beans (black, kidney, pinto, lima, white, soy, and many other varieties), lentils, and peas (chickpeas, split peas, black-eyed peas). In addition to protein and fiber, pulses contain many of the vitamins and minerals needed for healthy functioning of brain cells that are involved in memory.

▶ **Berries**—including strawberries, blueberries, bilberries, lingonberries, and raspberries—may reduce blood pressure and boost levels of healthy HDL cholesterol. Berries also may help prevent thickening of your carotid arteries, which supply blood to your brain. The MIND diet singles out berries as an ingredient because of the extensive research on berries' brain benefits. Berries' brain-protective power is thought to stem from their high content of phytonutrients called anthocyanins, compounds that give the fruits their vivid colors.

▶ **Carrots** contain phytonutrients called polyacetylenes that are being studied for possible cardiovascular benefits. These compounds seem to have anti-inflammatory properties that help keep blood cells from clumping together.

▶ **Cranberries** may protect the heart and blood vessels by reducing "bad" LDL cholesterol, combating oxidative stress, decreasing inflammation, improving the function of the lining of blood vessels, and increasing levels of nitric oxide, which dilates blood vessels.

▶ **Garlic** and other members of the *Allium* family, including shallots, leeks, and chives, are rich in sulfur compounds that may aid in preventing plaque buildup in arteries and controlling blood pressure and cholesterol.

▶ **Grapes** and grape juice may have brain benefits similar to those associated with berries. Grapes have been found to boost the brain's signaling functions, and Tufts researchers have reported that Concord grape juice reversed brain aging in rats.

▶ **Green leafy vegetables,** including kale, spinach, arugula, and collard and turnip greens, are high in the carotenoid lutein, which has been linked to a reduced risk of cognitive decline. They also provide folate and other nutrients that support cognitive functioning. One study of adults with an average age of 81 found that participants who consumed the most leafy greens (1.3 daily servings) had a slower rate of cognitive decline than participants who ate the least (0.1 daily servings). The green leafy vegetables the participants reported eating included spinach, kale, collards and other greens (one-half cup cooked equals one serving) and lettuce (one cup raw).

▶ **Onions,** another member of the *Allium* family, might help prevent platelets from sticking together, which could reduce the risk of atherosclerosis, stroke, and heart attack.

▶ **Oranges** contain compounds called limonoids, which have been linked with cholesterol benefits.

▶ **Pomegranate juice,** rich in antioxidants and phytonutrients, has been widely advertised for cardiovascular benefits, although supporting evidence is limited. A few small studies have reported blood pressure reductions of 6 to 7 percent in as little as two weeks of drinking a daily cup of pomegranate juice. Pomegranates are high in ellagic acid, a phytonutrient that acts as an antioxidant and may protect against heart disease. The juice is high in sugar and lacks fiber, so drink no more than one 8-ounce glass per day.

▶ **Tomatoes** (including tomato paste, sauce, and juice) may lower LDL cholesterol levels, and the potassium in tomatoes may help counter the blood pressure-raising effects of sodium. Lycopene, which gives tomatoes their rich, red color, has been associated with a lower risk of stroke in men. Lycopene also has been linked with improved cholesterol and triglyceride levels and a reduced risk of atherosclerosis.

Increase Your Produce Intake

Keeping in mind that more is better, it helps to have some basic goals when it comes to consuming vegetables and fruits. The U.S. Department of Agriculture advises that women over age 50 eat at least two cups of vegetables daily. Women between ages 19 and 50 should aim for two-and-a-half cups a day. Men over age 50 are advised to eat two-and-a-half cups of vegetables daily, and men between ages 19 and 50 should aim for at least three cups a day. (Count one cup of lettuce or leafy greens as a one-half cup serving.)

For fruit, women over 30 should consume one-and-a-half cups daily (two cups for women between ages 19 and 30), while adult men of all ages should aim for two cups per day.

There are a variety of creative ways to incorporate more veggies into your daily diet.

- Make stir-fry dishes with a modest amount of chicken or shrimp and a variety of tender-crisp vegetables.
- If you have an air fryer, mix veggies with a teaspoon or two of oil and "fry" them for a crispy side dish. Tender vegetables (broccoli, green beans, asparagus, cauliflower) take 10 minutes; firm vegetables (carrots, sweet potatoes, parsnips) take 15 minutes. Stir every five minutes for even cooking.
- Cook and purée vegetables and stir them into casseroles and soups.
- Finely chop spinach or kale and add to a pot of stew or a casserole.
- Stir diced, cooked vegetables into brown rice, quinoa, or other whole-grain side dishes.

- Stuff sandwiches with sliced cucumbers, mushrooms, and bell peppers, along with the traditional toppings of lettuce, tomatoes, and onions.

It's even easier to add fruits to your daily dietary pattern.

- Sprinkle berries or dried, no-sugar-added fruits such as raisins or apricots on your breakfast cereal.
- Blend bananas with low-fat yogurt and ice for a healthy smoothie; add fresh, frozen, or canned (unsweetened) pineapple, peaches, pears, cherries, or berries to get a double dose of fruit.
- Slice apples or pears onto a green salad.
- Keep a bowl of fresh fruit on your table or counter so it's easy to grab a piece for a snack.
- Choose fruit for a satisfyingly sweet dessert after dinner.

Go for Whole Grains

All grains start out as a seed or kernel that is surrounded by a protective husk. Once the husk is removed, three edible sections remain: the bran, germ, and endosperm. Whole grains are composed of all three of these sections, while refined grains contain only the endosperm; the bran and germ have been stripped away during processing. Since the bran and germ contain fiber, vitamins, minerals, and healthy fat, whole grains deliver more valuable nutrients to your brain and heart than refined grains. (Some "enriched" products made from grains, such as flour, have had some of these nutrients added back in.)

Whole grains include unprocessed versions of familiar foods, such as wheat and rice, as well as less-familiar grains that make tasty additions to your menus. Here are some whole grains to look for:

▶ **Amaranth:** An "ancient" grain that is high in protein.

▶ **Barley:** Look for whole or hulled barley.

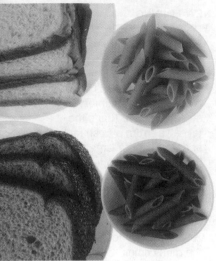
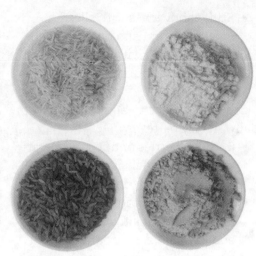

© Mitgirl | Dreamstime

An easy way to increase your whole-grain intake is to substitute whole-grain flour, rice, pasta, and bread in place of white flour, white rice, and pasta and bread made with refined white flour.

Pearled barley is not a whole grain, but it is still nutritious and easier to find and prepare.

▶ **Buckwheat:** Despite its name, this grain is unrelated to wheat. Buckwheat flour is a popular ingredient in pancakes.

▶ **Bulgur wheat:** These are wheat kernels that have been cooked, dried, and cracked. Bulgur wheat is the basis for tabouli (or tabbouleh), a popular Middle Eastern side dish that also contains fresh herbs.

▶ **Corn:** Cornmeal, polenta, grits, and other dried, ground forms of corn. Check the ingredients list; if you see the words "degermed" or "degerminated," it is not a whole grain. Popcorn is a whole grain, too.

▶ **Einkorn:** A variety of wheat.

▶ **Farro:** A variety of wheat that is also called "emmer." Look for whole farro; pearled farro is not a whole grain.

▶ **Kamut:** A variety of wheat.

▶ **Millet:** Varieties include pearl, foxtail, and finger millet.

▶ **Oats:** Oats, oatmeal, and oat groats are all whole grains.

▶ **Quinoa:** Quinoa is one of a handful of plant foods that supplies all the amino acids (notably lysine) in adequate amounts necessary for a "complete" protein. Technically, quinoa is a seed rather than a grain, but many of its properties are more similar to grains than seeds.

▶ **Rice:** Black, brown, red, and wild rice are whole grains; white rice is not.

▶ **Rye:** Look for whole rye and rye berries.

▶ **Spelt:** Look for whole spelt, a variety of wheat.

▶ **Wheat:** Look for whole wheat; wheat kernels that have not been cooked, cracked, or modified in any way are called "wheat berries."

Whole-Grain Health Benefits

The more studies researchers conduct on whole grains, the stronger the evidence of their health benefits becomes. One study examined whole-grain intake and mortality (death) rates; the researchers' analysis revealed that for every additional 50 grams of whole grains consumed, mortality rates decreased by 18 to 30 percent. The greatest benefit was associated with cardiovascular mortality, meaning that the more whole grains they consumed, the less likely they were to die from cardiovascular causes such as coronary artery disease, heart attack, or stroke. Similarly, another study found that people who consumed the most whole grains were 23 to 25 percent less likely to suffer a heart attack than those with the lowest intake of whole grains.

Eating whole grains also has been linked with better cholesterol numbers. Tufts researchers found that even people who are already taking statin medications to improve their cholesterol can achieve better results by also consuming more whole grains.

According to the Whole Grains Council, the benefits of including whole grains in your diet include:

- A reduced risk of stroke
- Healthier carotid arteries
- A decreased risk of heart disease
- Healthier blood pressure levels
- Better weight maintenance
- A lower risk of type 2 diabetes
- A reduced risk of colorectal cancer
- Less inflammation

Subbing in Whole Grains

Aim to make at least half of the grains you consume whole grains. Simple substitutions can make that goal easy to achieve: Choose whole-grain bread instead of white bread (including most Cuban, Italian, French, and sourdough varieties); brown or wild rice (or other whole grains such as quinoa, barley, or farro) in place of white rice; and whole-grain pasta instead of pasta made from semolina (a product made by milling durum wheat, which is specifically grown for pasta). In baking recipes, you can substitute whole-wheat flour for up to half of the all-purpose flour.

Expanding the variety of whole grains in your dietary pattern is another way to increase your consumption. Experiment with grains that are new to you; start by picking up a different type of whole grain each time you shop for groceries. Make cool summer salads with quinoa instead of pasta, and replace your cold breakfast cereal with a bowl of cooked amaranth or millet. Choosing popcorn instead of chips can make snack time healthier, as long as you skip the butter and limit the salt.

Just one serving of many whole-grain foods provides 16 grams of whole grains, including one slice of whole-grain bread or one-half cup of cooked brown rice, oatmeal, or whole-grain pasta. Check the ingredients list for terms such as "whole" (whole-wheat flour, whole oats) and look for the Whole Grain Stamp.

Don't be fooled by terms such as "multigrain" or "stoneground"—these words on product labels do not guarantee the product contains whole grains. High fiber content, though desirable, is not necessarily an indication of a whole-grain food. Also, when considering grain products such as breakfast cereals and granola bars, check the Nutrition Facts panel—many items that contain whole grains also are high in added sugars.

The Gluten-Free Fad

The only people who need to follow a gluten-free diet are those diagnosed with celiac disease or gluten sensitivity. They need to avoid all foods that contain gluten, including wheat (including wheat varieties like spelt, kamut, farro, and bulgur), barley, rye, and triticale. Fortunately, many grains are gluten-free, including rice, corn, amaranth, millet, and quinoa. Oats also are gluten-free, but some people with celiac disease react to a slightly different protein found in oats.

For everyone else, "going gluten-free" is a fad. It's smarter to stay focused on the proven nutritional benefits of grains than to be concerned about whether or not a grain contains gluten. Claims about wheat's supposed detrimental effects on cognition ("wheat brain") don't stand up to scientific scrutiny. All grains, including wheat, are key foods in both the DASH dietary plan and the Mediterranean-style diet, and research has linked both regimens to a lower risk of dementia.

The same goes for other notions linking wheat to abdominal fat ("wheat belly"). Scientific evidence does not support

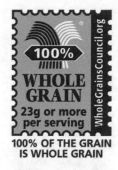

100% OF THE GRAIN IS WHOLE GRAIN

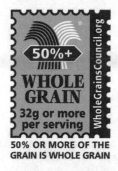

50% OR MORE OF THE GRAIN IS WHOLE GRAIN

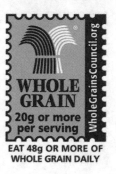

EAT 48g OR MORE OF WHOLE GRAIN DAILY

Finding Whole Grains

One way to make sure you're getting whole grains is to look for the whole-grain stamp developed by the Whole Grains Council, which many food manufacturers voluntarily use on their products. The Basic Stamp indicates that the product contains at least 8 grams, or half of a serving, of whole grains. The 100% Stamp indicates that all of the product's grain ingredients are whole grains, and that it contains at least 16 grams of whole grain per serving. No stamp? Check the label and ingredients list.

To make sure you're getting whole grains, look for these terms on the label and the ingredients list:

- whole grain [name of grain]
- whole wheat
- whole [other grain]
- stoneground whole [grain]

- brown rice
- oats, oatmeal (including instant oatmeal, old-fashioned oatmeal)
- wheat berries or wheatberries

These terms may or may NOT mean whole grain:

- wheat, or wheat flour
- semolina
- durum wheat
- organic flour

- stoneground
- multigrain (may describe several whole grains or several refined grains, or a mix of both)

Courtesy Oldways and the Whole Grains Council (wholegrainscouncil.org) claims that eating wheat is linked to greater abdominal adiposity, weight gain, or any other negative health effects. It's true that cutting out gluten-containing foods may temporarily lead to weight loss, but that will happen if you eliminate carbs, fat, or any other significant source of calories, including foods made with gluten-free grains, from your diet.

You're more likely to gain weight if you routinely choose processed foods that contain refined grains as well as added sugar and/or saturated fat (think cookies, pastries, doughnuts, cupcakes, and other pre-packaged baked goods). Conversely, eating sensible portions of nutrient-dense whole grains—whether or not they contain gluten—can help prevent weight gain, since their fiber content helps you feel full. And some research suggests that diets high in whole grains actually reduce the number of calories that are absorbed.

Nutrition in Nuts and Seeds

Nuts and seeds are rich in healthy unsaturated fats, and they are high in vitamin E, which has been linked to a lower risk of age-related cognitive decline. Additionally, they are a source of magnesium, a mineral linked to healthy blood pressure and fewer deaths from heart disease. They also provide plant protein and fiber.

Research has shown that people who include nuts in their diets have higher intakes of folate, beta-carotene, vitamin K, lutein plus zeaxanthin, phosphorus, copper, selenium, potassium, and zinc than people who don't eat nuts, even when they all consumed the same amount of calories. Nuts also have antioxidant and anti-inflammatory effects, which might have protective benefits for the heart and brain.

Multiple studies have found that eating nuts may lower the risk for heart disease and stroke. In one study, researchers found that eating any type of nuts five times a week was associated with a 14 percent reduction in cardiovascular events and a 20 percent reduction in coronary heart disease. Similar associations were seen when different types of nuts, including peanuts, were looked at separately.

A Tufts review of 61 prior studies found that nut intake was associated with lower total cholesterol, LDL cholesterol, and triglycerides. In another study, researchers calculated that people who consumed the most nuts had a 17 to 21 percent lower mortality risk than those who ate the fewest nuts.

Picking Nuts

When shopping for nuts, it's okay to go with whatever types taste best to you. Although there are slight nutritional differences among the many varieties of nuts, their similarities are more important.

Peanuts are actually legumes, but their nutritional profile closely resembles tree nuts. Studies have found health benefits from peanuts are similar to those associated with true tree nuts such as walnuts, almonds, pistachios, and cashews.

Nuts are nutrient dense, but they also are relatively high in calories, providing between 160 and 200 calories per one-ounce portion. Even though they are a concentrated source of calories, nuts don't appear to be linked to weight gain and might even help control weight. In a European study, people who consumed the most nuts gained slightly less weight and were less likely to become overweight than people whose diets contained the fewest nuts. Eating nuts may help with weight control because they contain protein and fiber, which may stave off hunger and help you resist empty-calorie snack foods.

Choices in Seeds

A rich source of healthy unsaturated fats and nutrients, seeds include flax, sesame, sunflower, pumpkin, chia, and hemp. Research suggests that flaxseed, which is high in the plant form of omega-3s, may benefit blood pressure. In one study, participants had significantly lower blood

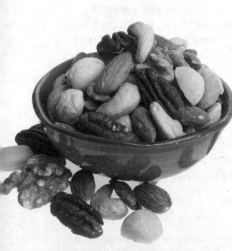

© Hein Teh | Dreamstime

Eating nuts several times a week may help lower your risk of stroke and heart disease.

pressure after they consumed 30 grams of milled flaxseed (about three heaping tablespoonsful) daily for six months. The researchers noted that the drops in some patients' blood pressure were similar to what may be achieved when taking blood pressure medication.

Seeds also provide fiber, protein, and a host of other valuable nutrients. Sprinkle them on oatmeal, into pancake and muffin batters, over salads, and into smoothies. Snack on sunflower or pumpkin seeds (watch the salt) instead of chips or crackers.

Why Eat Fish?

Experts advise eating more fish than most Americans typically do, with a recommendation of two meals of fish or other seafood per week. Although that advice generally includes a recommendation to choose varieties rich in omega-3 fatty acids, it's increasingly clear that the positive health effects of fish consumption go beyond any single ingredient. That may be why eating more fish is a recipe for better heart and brain health that can't be matched by simply popping fish-oil pills.

Fish is rich in protein and other important nutrients, and it's relatively low in calories if it's prepared healthfully—without frying, breading, globs of butter, or creamy sauces. Steaming, broiling, grilling, baking, and poaching with little or no added fat will best preserve the beneficial nutrients in fish without adding ingredients you don't need. Since overfishing can decimate fish populations, select fish that are sustainably grown and harvested.

Omega-3s and Your Heart

Evidence linking cardiovascular benefits with the omega-3 fatty acids found in fish is extensive. Varieties higher in omega-3 fatty acids include salmon (wild and sockeye), trout, herring, sardines, and mackerel. While these varieties are highly recommended, if you don't like them, try milder fish such as tilapia, cod, and other whitefish; although they are lower in omega-3s, substituting any type of fish for fried chicken, ribs, or steak represents a positive trade-off.

An analysis of 19 studies involving 45,637 participants in 16 countries provides the most comprehensive picture to date of how omega-3 fats may influence heart disease. People with the highest blood levels of omega-3s from seafood as well as plants had about a 25 percent lower risk of fatal heart attack, compared to people with the lowest levels.

Other studies have shown that intake of omega-3 fatty acids is associated with reduced risk of arrhythmias (abnormal heartbeat), decreased triglyceride levels, and slower growth of atherosclerotic plaque.

Skip the Fish Oil Pills. If you're taking fish oil pills instead of eating fish to protect your heart, a meta-analysis published in 2018 suggests you might be wasting your money. The analysis of 10 large randomized trials lasting at least one year found that fish oil supplements were not associated with a significantly reduced risk of death from coronary heart disease (CHD), any CHD events, or major vascular events such as stroke, and other studies have found little or no evidence linking fish oil supplements with better heart health.

However, if you do choose to take a fish oil supplement (or any other type), check if the supplement has been tested and verified by an agency such as the U.S. Pharmacopeia. Since supplements are not regulated by any government agency, there's no guarantee that what's on the label is actually in the bottle. And if you take any medications, get your doctor's approval before taking any supplement; some may interact with medications, causing problematic side effects or changing the effectiveness of the drug.

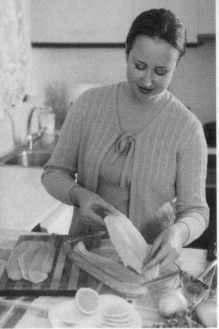
© Iakov Filimonov | Dreamstime

The healthiest cooking methods for fish are baking, broiling, poaching, and grilling with a small amount of healthy fat, such as olive, canola, or soybean oil.

Brain Benefits from Fish

Eating fish—especially varieties higher in omega-3s—also seems to be good for the brain. One study found that the brains of people with high blood levels of omega-3s showed greater blood flow in areas of the brain involved in memory and learning, and the people also scored higher on tests of cognitive function than people with lower blood levels of omega-3s.

Another study used MRI scans to compare the brain volumes of those who ate more fish with non-fish eaters: The scans revealed that people who ate broiled or baked fish, but not fried fish, on a weekly basis had greater volumes of gray matter in the brain's frontal and temporal lobes, as well as in the hippocampus, an area that plays a key role in memory.

Previously, Tufts researchers who studied brain function and fish consumption reported that people who ate the most fish, as well as those with higher blood levels of the omega-3 fat DHA, were at sharply lower risk of dementia and Alzheimer's disease than people who ate less or no fish.

The omega-3 fatty acids in fish also may protect the brain from infarcts (tissue damaged by a lack of blood flow) that can lead to impaired thinking skills, dementia, and full-blown stroke.

Mercury Worries. If concerns about mercury in seafood have kept you from consuming more fish, an unusual study has good news. Researchers found that older adults who ate more seafood had higher brain levels of mercury—but the higher levels were not associated with a higher risk of dementia. (Mercury in seafood is nonetheless a concern for children, pregnant women, women who might become pregnant, and nursing mothers because high mercury levels can harm a fetus or a child's nervous system.) The FDA says levels of PCBs (toxic chemicals that settle into water and soil) in fish also are well below safety limits, but, if you're concerned, select wild rather than farm-raised fish.

Fresh, Frozen, or Canned?

People who don't live near the coast and who don't have ready access to fish markets can still enjoy the health benefits of seafood. If your supermarket's fresh-fish selection is meager, don't hesitate to turn to the freezer section. (Often, much of what's displayed as "fresh" fish was previously frozen, anyway.) Shop for fish labeled "Frozen-at-Sea" (FAS), which is caught by crews on ships that operate like floating processing plants. Flash-frozen the same day they're caught, these fish often retain more nutrients than fish that is never frozen but is kept on ice for a week or more.

Canned fish is another good option. Canned sardines and salmon are generally sustainable choices; canned tuna, while controversial, typically includes sustainable, pole-caught albacore or skipjack varieties (check the label).

The varieties of fish that are canned or packaged in handy pouches are often the same fish that are high in omega-3s, notably salmon and albacore ("white") tuna. Omega-3s aren't destroyed in the canning process, so you're not sacrificing heart-brain health for convenience.

Beverages from Plants: Tea and Coffee

Drinking tea and coffee isn't quite like eating a serving of vegetables, but these popular beverages are packed with beneficial phytonutrients called flavonoids—much like other plant foods. Both beverages also have been associated with health benefits.

Drinking tea has been associated with lower blood pressure, reduced risk of heart attacks, and improved cholesterol levels. Other research suggests that compounds in tea can repair injuries to the brain's neurons associated with aging. Findings from one study suggested that green tea may improve the connectivity between parts of the brain involved in tasks of working memory.

Scientists have paid special attention to a phytonutrient called epicatechin, which is found in tea as well as in cocoa and apples. One study reported that, among older men who had cardiovascular disease at the study's outset, an epicatechin intake that was roughly equivalent to the amount in one cup of brewed green tea was associated with a 46 percent lower risk of death from cardiovascular disease during a 25-year follow-up period.

Coffee Is Good for You

As for coffee, forget those warnings that it's bad for you. The Dietary Guidelines Advisory Committee concluded that drinking three to five cups a day of coffee (up to about 400 milligrams of caffeine) was associated with minimal health risks and may actually have benefits.

One large study reported that people drinking three to five cups of coffee daily were 41 percent less likely to have calcium buildup in their coronary arteries than non-coffee drinkers. The presence of coronary artery calcium (CAC) is an early indicator of heart disease. Coffee drinkers at all levels of consumption were less likely to have CAC than non-coffee drinkers.

In another study, drinking coffee—both regular and decaf—was linked to a reduced risk of death from cardiovascular disease. Other researchers have linked coffee intake to lower risks of type 2 diabetes and cardiovascular disease.

Even beyond the short-term mental lift associated with caffeine, coffee appears to have beneficial effects on brain function. In one study, men who consumed three cups of coffee a day suffered significantly less cognitive decline over 10 years compared to non-coffee drinkers. Another study reported that older women who drank at least three cups of coffee daily were less likely to develop problems with memory than those who drank less coffee.

However, keep in mind that dosing your coffee (or tea) with sugar, cream, and/or various sweet flavorings can more than outweigh the beverages' benefits.

Caffeine Questions. Both regular tea and coffee contain the stimulant caffeine. Since caffeine's effects include increasing the heart rate and boosting blood flow, concerns have arisen that too much caffeine might harm the heart or cause disturbances in heart rhythm. However, research in recent years has laid these concerns to rest.

An average cup of black tea contains less caffeine than coffee, and green tea contains even less caffeine than black tea; the longer and stronger the brew, the higher the caffeine content. If you experience unpleasant side effects such as nervousness, insomnia, or upset stomach from caffeine consumption, consider decaffeinated beverages, which, according to multiple studies, have similar benefits as regular tea and coffee.

Is Chocolate A Health Food?

Another food long considered an unhealthy indulgence—chocolate—has gotten a healthier reputation lately. Cocoa, the key ingredient in chocolate, contains phytonutrients called flavonoids, which have been associated with lower blood pressure and improved blood flow throughout the circulatory system.

Most studies have looked at the flavonoids in dark chocolate for heart benefits. However, some research also has found an association between milk-chocolate consumption and reduced

NEW FINDING

Coffee, Tea May Reduce Arrhythmia Risk

People with atrial fibrillation (A-fib) and other heart arrhythmias (irregular heartbeats) that increase stroke risk don't need to avoid coffee and tea. Not only are moderate amounts safe—research also suggests coffee and tea may even reduce arrhythmia frequency. A comprehensive review of studies on caffeinated beverages and heart rhythm found no evidence that drinking moderate amounts of coffee or tea triggered A-fib or other arrhythmias. Most of the studies reviewed also showed a reduced frequency of arrhythmias; regular coffee drinkers, for example, had a 6 percent reduction in A-fib frequency and a 13 percent lower risk of incident A-fib.

However, energy drinks that contain high levels of caffeine were found to be a potential trigger for arrhythmia. Researchers advised that patients with pre-existing heart conditions avoid energy drinks.

JACC: Clinical Electrophysiology, April 2018

Moderate Drinking Safest for Brain

Findings from a large study suggest that too much—or too little—alcohol consumption is associated with greater risk of dementia.

In the study, people who consumed one to 14 standard drinks per week (considered a moderate amount) had the lowest risk of dementia, while those who abstained from alcohol completely were at 47 percent greater risk. And every seven-drink increase in weekly consumption (for example, 21 drinks per week compared to 14 drinks per week) was linked to a 17 percent greater dementia risk. People with a high score on a measure of alcohol dependence had more than twice the rate of dementia.

Researchers also found that non-drinkers who did not have cardiometabolic disease (a combination of factors involving blood sugar, belly fat, cholesterol, and blood pressure) were at lower risk of dementia than non-drinkers with the disease, suggesting that factors that affect heart health also affect brain health.

BMJ, Aug. 1, 2018

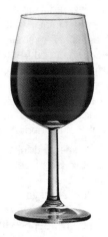

© Pluypen | Dreamstime

Five ounces of wine counts as one drink.

What Counts as One Drink?

Your alcoholic drinks might actually be more generous than one "drink," as defined by the government. One standard drink contains approximately 14 grams of alcohol. Examples include:

- 12 fluid ounces regular beer
- 8–9 fluid ounces malt liquor
- 5 fluid ounces wine
- 1.5 fluid ounces 80-proof spirits, such as whiskey, gin, and rum

risks of heart disease, stroke, and death from cardiovascular causes.

Other findings have suggested that moderate chocolate consumption doesn't harm, and may even help, cholesterol levels. Dark chocolate consumption has been linked to reductions in both total cholesterol and LDL cholesterol.

One study reported that, compared with eating chocolate less than once a month, moderate chocolate intake was associated with a 10 to 20 percent decreased risk of being diagnosed with atrial fibrillation ("A-fib," the most common type of irregular heartbeat). For women, the benefits associated with chocolate plateaued at one serving a week. For men, benefits started to plateau at six servings a week.

Chocolate on the Brain. Research also has linked consumption of dark chocolate and cocoa with improved cognition among people who have mild cognitive impairment, as well as improved function in areas of the brain important to memory. Patients with a condition called impaired neurovascular coupling experienced improved blood flow to the brain, as well as better cognitive scores, after drinking two cups of cocoa daily.

When choosing chocolate and cocoa, try to avoid products that are "Dutch-processed" or "alkalized." These terms indicate that the cacao beans were processed with alkali, which decreases the phytonutrient content. Also, keep your portions modest to avoid extra calories and saturated fat.

Wine and Your Heart

The health benefits of alcoholic beverages, notably red wine, are controversial. Resveratrol, a substance found in red wine and grapes, has been associated with better scores on memory tests and greater functional connectivity in the brain. Most studies, however, have used amounts of resveratrol far in excess of what you would obtain from a glass or two of red wine.

Other research has suggested that drinking red wine may boost the healthy effects of omega-3 fatty acids found in fish. This finding may help explain some of the cardiovascular benefits of the Mediterranean-style diet, which incorporates both fish and wine.

Drinking Downsides. Keep in mind that wine, like all alcoholic beverages, should be consumed in moderation only, defined as no more than one alcoholic drink daily for women and two for men. (A recent observational study suggests that even those standard recommendations may be too high, based on increasing mortality risk with intakes above five or six drinks per week.)

Drinking excessively can increase your risk for accidents, as well as high blood pressure, stroke, and other diseases. Even small amounts of alcohol appear to increase the risk of breast and other cancers. Overdoing it also can be bad for your brain: Middle-age men who averaged two-and-a-half or more drinks daily showed faster 10-year declines in cognitive function than did lighter drinkers.

If you don't drink alcohol, experts advise that the possible benefits are not enough reason to start drinking. If you don't like wine or choose not to drink alcohol, red grape juice contains the same phytonutrients as red wine, which help improve blood vessel health and protect against high blood pressure.

Be Skeptical of Supplement Claims

Just as it's better to eat fish than to rely on fish oil pills, it's smart to be skeptical of any supplement promising heart and brain benefits: Pills can't compare with the nutrition you get from consuming whole foods. The nutrients in foods work together synergistically in ways that provide more benefits than if you were to consume them individually. Studies of individual vitamins and minerals in pill form have repeatedly failed to duplicate the benefits of consuming those same vitamins and minerals in food.

Some people say they take dietary supplements as "insurance" against nutritional shortfalls in their diets, and it's true that a few nutrients in supplement form can be beneficial. For example, if your vitamin B_{12} or vitamin D level is low, your doctor may recommend supplementation.

Other so-called "supplements" don't truly supplement any substances your body requires. Ginkgo biloba, for example, continues to be sold as a "brain-boosting" supplement, but the evidence for its benefits is extremely limited. The same holds for the widely advertised "jellyfish protein" purported to improve short-term memory.

If you take a daily multivitamin "just in case," don't expect to reap any heart benefits right away, if ever. A study of a group of male physicians reported an association between taking a multivitamin for at least 20 years and a lower risk of major cardiovascular events, compared to not taking a multivitamin—but fewer years of multivitamin

use were not linked with lower risks. Other factors may help account for the risk reduction, in any case: Long-term supplement users have other lifestyle behaviors associated with a lower risk of cardiovascular disease.

Buyer Beware

Keep in mind that products sold as "dietary supplements" aren't subject to the same U.S. Food & Drug Administration regulations as are drugs and foods. Analyses of numerous supplements have shown that some don't contain the amount of the active ingredient that the label claims (the amount may be higher or lower), and some contain ingredients not listed on the label, including potentially harmful lead, mercury, pesticides, and other toxic materials.

Another reason for caution is that supplements can interact with medications you may be taking. For example, ginseng, garlic, feverfew, fish oil, and several other supplements may interfere with the action of warfarin (Coumadin), a medication taken by millions of Americans.

Always discuss supplementation with your doctor, who can help determine if you are deficient in any essential nutrients and, if so, what type and dosage of supplement is best for you. If you do take supplements, make sure to tell your doctor so he or she can evaluate the risks of possible interactions with any medications you take.

NEW FINDING

Most Supplements Don't Deliver

If you're concerned about your heart and how your cardiovascular health affects your brain, you can mostly skip the supplements aisle. A new review of 179 randomized controlled trials concludes that most commonly used vitamin and mineral supplements don't prevent cardiovascular disease, events, or all-cause mortality. The review found no consistent cardiovascular benefit, including stroke prevention, from multivitamins or supplements of vitamin D, calcium, vitamin C, beta-carotene, or selenium.

Positive findings for supplements included a link between B vitamins (folic acid, B_6, B_{12}) and lower stroke risk. And one Chinese study found that taking folic acid was tied to lower cardiovascular risks. However, food is not fortified with folic acid in China as it is in North America, where consumers should be cautious about supplemental folic acid.

Journal of the American College of Cardiology, June 2018

USP Verified Mark

One way to be sure a supplement contains what the label promises is to look for this seal. The USP mark indicates that the supplement has been tested by the U.S. Pharmacopeia and found to contain the ingredients on the label in the declared strengths and amounts. Supplements that are USP verified also have been found to be free of potentially harmful contaminants, and have been created in sanitary conditions and by well-controlled processes in accordance with FDA and USP Good Manufacturing Practices.

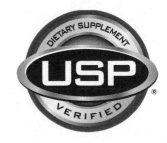

A typical fast-food meal is high in saturated fat, sodium, and sugar—all of which can harm, rather than help, your heart and brain.

4 Nutrition Negatives

As we saw in the previous chapter, scientific evidence supports plenty of healthy choices for your heart and brain that you can enjoy as part of your healthy dietary pattern. Just as smart dietary choices can help protect your heart and brain, however, poor dietary decisions can increase your risk for cardiovascular disease and dementia. While small amounts of most dietary "don'ts" generally won't cause serious harm, they should be considered indulgences enjoyed as an occasional treat. For many Americans, unfortunately, "don'ts" such as foods high in sodium or saturated fat, and soft drinks and sweets loaded with added sugars, are mainstays of their daily diets.

Be Smart About Fats

We've already seen how the "low-fat" craze had unintended weight-gain consequences, and that it's okay to consume unsaturated fats. Other types of dietary fat, however, should be limited because of how they affect cholesterol levels in your blood (serum cholesterol). Unhealthy cholesterol levels, in turn, can have a damaging effect on your cardiovascular system as well as your brain.

Your genes partly determine whether your body produces too much unhealthy LDL cholesterol or effectively removes excess serum cholesterol from your blood. But your diet also can impact your LDL cholesterol and triglyceride levels (a type of fat in the bloodstream that, when elevated, increases heart disease risk). Research on the complex effects of fats from food on fats in your bloodstream is ongoing, but the primary dietary culprits that contribute to unhealthy cholesterol levels seem to be saturated fat and trans fat.

Limit Saturated Fat

The main sources of saturated fat in the U.S. diet are cheese, pizza, desserts, and skin-on chicken and chicken dishes (even though poultry has less saturated fat than most cuts of beef, we eat more of it). Other sources of saturated fat include butter, lard, whole milk, and fatty cuts of beef and pork.

Chemically speaking, saturated fats are fat molecules that have no double bonds between carbon molecules because they are "saturated" with hydrogen atoms. (Unsaturated fats have at least one location that is not occupied by a hydrogen atom.) Saturated fats are typically solid at room temperature (like butter or lard).

Scientists believe that saturated fat is the chief dietary contributor to unhealthy serum cholesterol levels. In its latest scientific advisory on the subject, the American Heart Association reaffirmed that saturated fat raises unhealthy LDL cholesterol levels.

However, scientists are learning that not all forms of saturated fat affect the body in the same way or to the same degree: Recent research suggests that the fat in dairy products may be less harmful than that from other sources.

Target Numbers. The current *Dietary Guidelines for Americans (DGA)* recommend getting less than 10 percent of your daily calories from saturated fat. For a person who consumes 2,000 calories per day, that works out to 20 grams or less. For people who have high LDL cholesterol, the American Heart Association recommends getting a maximum of 6 percent of total calories from saturated fat; that's no more than 12 grams of saturated fat if you're eating 2,000 calories a day. To put this in perspective, a grilled, 8-ounce rib-eye steak has about 8 grams of saturated fat (even after trimming the external fat), a baked potato with two teaspoons of butter and two tablespoons of sour cream has 7 grams of saturated fat, and a cup of vanilla ice cream has 9 grams of saturated fat.

Studies have shown that replacing saturated fat with polyunsaturated fat found in plant foods, such as vegetable oils, avocados, nuts, and seeds, is an effective way to improve cardiovascular health. Another healthy choice is monounsaturated fat; one source is olive oil, a key ingredient in the Mediterranean-style diet. All oils contain a mixture of saturated and unsaturated fats, so the goal is to choose those relatively low in saturated fat; these include most vegetable oils, with the exception of palm, palm kernel, and coconut oils, which are high in saturated fat.

Cut Back on Fatty Meats. Meat is a major source of saturated fat for carnivorous Americans, though not all meats are equally high in saturated fat. Meats (including beef, pork, and lamb) that are highest in saturated fat have the most total fat. Often, you can identify meat that's high in saturated fat just by looking at it: If you see a lot of "marbling"—streaks and specks of fat throughout the meat—and/or there's a lot of fat on the edges, it's high in saturated fat.

Choose lean cuts of meat (look for the words "round" and "loin," such as bottom round roast, pork tenderloin, or top sirloin), and avoid cuts like porterhouse, T-bone, NY strip, and ribeye. When buying ground beef or pork, select products that are 95-percent-lean. And avoid processed and cured meats, including most bacon, sausage, ham, deli meats, and hot dogs, which are high in saturated fat as

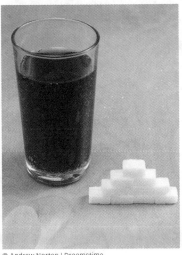

© Andrew Norton | Dreamstime

Many 12-ounce soft drinks contain about 10 teaspoons of sugar.

well as sodium. The World Health Organization has classified processed meats as probable carcinogens, meaning they probably cause cancer. Eating an average of 50 grams (about 1.8 ounces) of processed meat per day has been linked to an 18 percent increased risk of colorectal cancer.

Cutting your consumption of beef and pork can have clear benefits. One study found that replacing one serving of red meat daily with a serving of fish, low-fat dairy, or nuts may cut heart disease risk by up to 30 percent.

Poultry also can be high in saturated fat. When cooking or eating poultry, choose skinless options or throw away the skin, which contains the most saturated fat. Also, breast meat has less saturated fat than thigh or leg meat.

No More Trans Fat

The fat that's worst for your heart and brain is industrially produced (man-made) trans fat found in partially hydrogenated oils (PHOs). This fat raises LDL cholesterol and lowers "good" HDL cholesterol. Food manufacturers added PHOs to all types of highly processed foods, ranging from crackers and snack cakes to coffee creamers and frostings.

Based on the evidence of trans fat's harmful effects, the U.S. Food & Drug Administration banned PHOs, which were removed from most food products by 2018. However, the compliance date for a few products was extended until 2020. If in doubt, check ingredients on packages of processed foods for the term "partially hydrogenated oil."

Don't Count on Coconut Oil

Although it is high in saturated fat, coconut oil has been touted as a "superfood" by some who say the saturated fat in coconuts, lauric acid, has different properties than the saturated fat found in animal foods. Advocates claim that coconut oil reduces obesity and protects the brain.

A few small studies that examined the effects of consuming pure lauric acid have shown a modest reduction in body weight, but studies in which actual coconut oil (which is 44 percent lauric acid) was used did not achieve similar results. In short, no studies have conclusively shown that coconut oil provides heart or brain benefits, especially with long-term use.

Most health experts advise using vegetable oils such as olive, canola, soybean, and corn oils that are high in unsaturated fat rather than coconut oil. That said, occasional use of small amounts of coconut oil is unlikely to cause health problems—just don't count on coconut oil to improve your health.

Cut Down on Sodium

In and of itself, sodium is not unhealthy; in fact, sodium is essential for regulating blood pressure and helping your muscles and nerves function normally. It's the excessive sodium found in the typical "Western" diet that has been linked to high blood pressure. Many people with hypertension can lower their blood pressure by limiting their intake of sodium chloride—the chemical name for salt.

What's the link between sodium and blood pressure? When you consume too much sodium, your body retains extra water, which increases blood volume and blood pressure in your circulatory system. In addition to its effects on blood pressure, sodium also may directly increase the risk of cardiovascular disease by decreasing the flexibility of blood vessels and hardening cells in the heart.

How much sodium is too much remains controversial. The DGA recommends a 2,300-milligram (mg) sodium maximum, and the American Heart Association advises that, for most adults, a 1,500-mg limit is ideal. Whatever the exact recommendation, experts advise that most people would benefit by cutting down on their intake. About

90 percent of Americans consume too much sodium, according to the American Heart Association.

Salt-Reduction Strategies

An estimated 80 percent of the sodium in the American diet comes from processed, packaged, and restaurant foods, rather than being added during cooking or at the table. If you eat out frequently, cooking more meals at home is one strategy that will reduce your sodium intake while also improving your overall dietary quality. When you opt for the convenience of canned products such as beans and tomatoes, choose no-salt-added or low-sodium products, or drain and rinse them to remove excess sodium.

Use more herbs and spices and less salt in the foods you prepare. In fact, spicing things up actually might reduce your salt cravings: A large Chinese study reported that people with a penchant for spicier foods preferred less salt, and they consumed less total sodium and had lower blood pressures than people who used fewer seasonings and more salt. Adding a few splashes of lime or lemon juice or vinegar also can make low-sodium foods taste less bland.

Avoid Added Sugar

Diets high in added sugar have been linked to higher blood pressure, lower HDL cholesterol levels, elevated triglyceride levels, weight gain, and obesity, which are all linked to a greater risk of cardiovascular disease.

Many studies have provided evidence for the connection between added sugar and cardiovascular disease. In one study, men who reported drinking two or more servings daily of soft drinks or sweetened juice drinks were 23 percent more likely to develop heart failure than men who drank no sweetened beverages. In another study, participants who drank an average of three sugary beverages a week gained 7.4 percent more visceral fat than those who consumed less than one sugary drink a month. Visceral fat, which surrounds the organs in the abdomen, is associated with higher risks of heart disease and high blood pressure.

The DGA calls for limiting added sugars to fewer than 10 percent of total calories per day. In a 2,000-calorie daily diet, that means no more than 200 calories from added sugars—about 12 teaspoons of sugar, or about the amount in one regular 16-ounce soft drink. (One teaspoon of sugar has 16 calories and is the equivalent of 4 grams.)

Why the focus on "added" sugar? Although all sugars affect the body similarly, naturally occurring sugars in foods are part of a package that also includes healthy nutrients, such as vitamins, minerals, and/or fiber. Naturally occurring sugars in milk and fruit don't count toward the recommended limit.

Sources of Sugar

You can start reducing your added-sugar intake by skipping sugary sodas and other drinks. Nearly half of the added sugar consumed by Americans comes from sodas, sports drinks, and fruit drinks. And don't overlook those "gourmet" tea and coffee drinks—that iced chai or mocha frappuccino may contain as much as 15 teaspoons of added sugar.

Some foods are surprising sources of sugar, too. An estimated 75 percent of packaged foods purchased in the U.S. contain added sugar. Candy and desserts are obvious culprits, but sugar also is added to ketchup, salad dressings, breads, bagels, and baked beans.

Identifying added sugars in your foods and beverages can be tricky. The updated Nutrition Facts label that's already rolling out on some packages requires a line for added sugars that's separate from the line for total sugars. If a food's Nutrition Facts label doesn't yet list added sugars, check ingredient lists for terms indicating sugar of any type.

"Sneaky" Sugar

If you see the word "sugar" or "syrup" in a food's ingredients list, it contains added sugar. However, there also are many types of sugar with many different names that are not easily identified as sugar. All of these ingredients are forms of added sugar:

- Agave nectar
- Cane crystals
- Corn sweetener
- Crystalline fructose
- Dextrose
- Evaporated cane juice
- Fructose
- Fruit juice concentrate
- Glucose
- Honey
- Maltose
- Molasses
- Sucrose

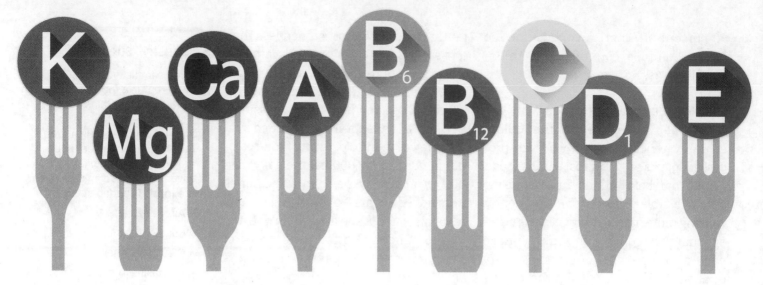

© Mast3r | Dreamstime

Your heart and brain require adequate amounts of several vitamins and minerals to function optimally.

5 The Nutrients You Need

Eating foods that fit into a healthy dietary pattern while limiting those that don't is the surest way to obtain the nutrients you need for your heart and brain. All nutritious foods contain a mix of nutrients, so you shouldn't look at any one food as a "magic bullet" for this vitamin or that mineral.

Nonetheless, in the typical American diet, it is true that some specific nutrients are often lacking. Experts say American adults don't consume enough vitamin D, potassium, fiber, and calcium. Each of these nutrients plays a role in the health of your heart and brain.

Vitamin D deficiency has been associated with a wide range of chronic conditions, including cardiovascular disease and dementia. Potassium can help control high blood pressure, an important risk factor for stroke. Dietary fiber helps reduce the risk of cardiovascular disease, among other benefits. In addition to the key role it plays in bone health, calcium also is needed for effective constriction and dilation of blood vessels, nerve transmission, and muscle contraction.

These nutrients, as well as some of the other nutrients that are most critical to your heart and brain, are discussed in this chapter.

Vitamin D

It's important to get enough vitamin D to avoid deficiency, but hopes that extra vitamin D might have significant heart or brain benefits have not been supported by rigorous clinical trials. It may be that vitamin D has what scientists call a "threshold" effect. It's important to get 100 percent of what's needed, and there are clear benefits to avoiding deficiency—but intakes of vitamin D above a certain threshold may have few or no additional benefits.

What D Does

We know that vitamin D plays an important role in various functions throughout the body. Many studies support the idea that people with adequate vitamin D levels enjoy protective benefits, and that there are risks associated with deficiency.

One study reported that supplements of vitamin D and calcium might modestly improve your cholesterol numbers. Participants taking supplements that contained 1,000 milligrams of calcium plus 400 IU of vitamin D had lower levels of unhealthy LDL cholesterol and triglycerides and higher levels of healthy HDL cholesterol, compared to participants who took a placebo.

Low levels of vitamin D also have been linked to cognitive decline and dementia. In a Tufts study of nearly 1,100 seniors, those with higher levels of vitamin D performed better on tests of executive function, such as planning, organizing, and thinking abstractly. And in a review of 25 prior studies, 18 of the studies showed that individuals with low vitamin D levels did worse on tests of cognitive functioning or were more likely to develop dementia than individuals with higher levels of vitamin D.

Getting Enough

The authoritative advice of the Institute of Medicine (IOM) calls for adults younger than age 70 to aim for a daily intake of vitamin D of 600 IU (International Units), while those older than 70 need 800 IU. Bess Dawson-Hughes, MD, director of Tufts' HNRCA Bone Metabolism Laboratory, says, "Complying with the Institute of Medicine's recommended doses should provide the best protection, and going overboard is to be avoided."

Achieving those targets may be challenging, however. Vitamin D is called the "sunshine vitamin" because the skin naturally makes vitamin D when exposed to sunlight. But many people lack the sun exposure necessary for their bodies to make vitamin D, and residents in the northern half of the U.S. are unable to produce enough vitamin D in the winter months because the sun's UV index is too low. Age also plays a role; as you get older, your body does not produce as much vitamin D. And a limited number of foods contain vitamin D, which can make it difficult to get adequate amounts from your diet alone.

People who are at risk of vitamin D deficiency include elderly and disabled people who reside in health-care facilities, people with very dark skin, people with a high percentage of body fat, and people who always cover up or use

Map of Winter Vitamin D Deficiency

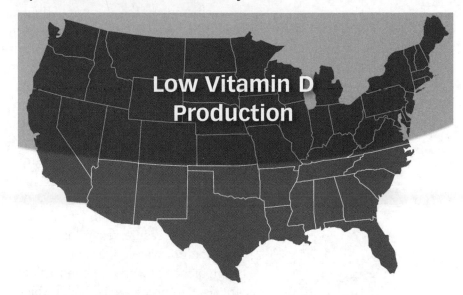

© Deskcube | Dreamstime

It's not just the northernmost states that are at risk of vitamin D deficiency in the winter; it's the northern half of the U.S., which includes Virginia, Kentucky, Missouri, Colorado, Utah, most of Nevada, and half of California.

sunscreen when outdoors. Gastrointestinal disorders and some medications can affect how well vitamin D is absorbed and how quickly it is broken down. People who have a vitamin D deficiency may need to boost their intake with supplements—a simple blood test can measure your vitamin D level.

Sources of Vitamin D

Here are the three sources of vitamin D:

- **Foods, including salmon,** swordfish, mackerel, sardines, halibut, flounder, rainbow trout, tuna, eggs, mushrooms (especially those exposed to ultraviolet light during growing)
- **Foods fortified with vitamin D,** including many brands of milk, yogurt, ready-to-eat cereals, orange juice, non-dairy milk, tofu (check the label to see if vitamin D has been added)
- **Exposing your skin to direct sunlight for short periods of time a few times a week,** especially in summer months. However, if you are at high risk of or have had skin cancer and your dermatologist has advised against sun exposure, follow your doctor's advice, and never stay in the sun for long periods without using sunscreen.

Potassium

Too much sodium raises your blood pressure by increasing the amount of fluid in your blood vessels, whereas potassium balances sodium's effects and helps lower your blood pressure by removing excess fluid. Observational studies consistently show that diets with an abundance of foods rich in potassium, as well as magnesium and other minerals, are associated with lower blood pressure.

In addition, numerous studies have demonstrated a relationship between higher dietary potassium intake and lower blood pressure, regardless of how much sodium was consumed.

High blood pressure is the most significant risk factor for stroke, making blood pressure control important for both heart and brain. In one study of more than 180,000 women, combined intake of potassium, magnesium, and calcium was associated with lower stroke risk. Women whose diets were highest in these minerals were 28 percent less likely to suffer any kind of stroke, and women with the highest potassium intake had an 11 percent lower risk of stroke.

Other research has shown that postmenopausal women who consumed the most potassium were 12 percent less likely to suffer a stroke of any kind than those who consumed the least potassium.

Potassium Targets

The Adequate Intake (AI) for adults is 4,700 milligrams of potassium daily, but average consumption is far below that, with one survey finding that adult men are consuming an average of only 3,100 milligrams of potassium per day and adult women are consuming about 2,400 milligrams each day.

Many potassium-rich foods are fruits and vegetables. Tufts expert Alice H. Lichtenstein, DSc, notes, "It is fortunate that good sources of potassium include all the types of foods that should be encouraged. Hence, even small steps toward improving the overall quality of the diet will likely result in an increase in potassium intake."

In addition to getting potassium from dietary sources, you can decrease your salt intake by switching to a salt substitute that contains potassium.

For most people, it's better to get potassium from foods than from potassium supplements. In fact, you should consume a potassium supplement only under the direction and supervision of your physician. Your body tightly regulates potassium levels in your blood, and supplementation may lead to hyperkalemia (high potassium), which can be just as dangerous as very low levels of potassium.

Sources of Potassium

As noted before, many fruits and vegetables are good sources of potassium, but grains, fish, and dairy also can help you meet your potassium target.

- **Vegetables:** Sweet potatoes, broccoli, avocados, beets, Brussels sprouts, tomatoes/tomato juice, potatoes, leafy greens, beans, eggplant
- **Fruits:** Bananas, cantaloupe, honeydew, nectarines, oranges/orange juice, peaches, prunes/prune juice
- **Fish:** Tuna, halibut, cod, trout
- **Dairy:** Milk, yogurt
- **Grains:** Brown rice, wild rice, oats

Other Nutrients That Affect Blood Pressure

As noted, other minerals, including magnesium and calcium, have been linked with lower blood pressure. Tufts researchers also have linked higher magnesium intake to reduced calcification in the coronary arteries. However, it's estimated that 70 to 80 percent of U.S. adults fail to get the recommended intake of magnesium (for adults ages 31 and older, 420 milligrams for men and 320 milligrams for women).

Besides its well-known bone-building benefits, dietary calcium also may pro-

---

NEW FINDING

Supplements Disappoint for Heart Protection

Don't count on vitamin D or fish oil pills to protect your heart. That's the conclusion of the VITAL study, which compared supplements to placebos among almost 13,000 participants over more than five years. No significant difference in major cardiovascular events was seen between people receiving vitamin D pills (2,000 IU daily) versus a control group.

Similarly, people randomly assigned to take fish oil pills (1,000 milligrams daily) suffered about the same number of major cardiovascular events as those in the control group.

New England Journal of Medicine, Nov. 10, 2018

mote healthy blood pressure levels. The recommended daily intake of calcium is 1,000 milligrams for women between ages 19 and 50 and for men between ages 19 and 70. Women age 51 and older and men age 71 and older are advised to get 1,200 milligrams of calcium daily.

Sources of Magnesium and Calcium

▶ **Magnesium:** Quinoa, brown rice, teff, and other whole grains, soymilk and soy yogurt, bran cereal, pumpkin and sesame seeds, nuts, Swiss chard, spinach, beans, bananas, green peas

▶ **Calcium:** Milk, yogurt, and other dairy products, beans, canned salmon and sardines (with bones), collard and turnip greens, spinach, soybeans, kale, and fortified cereals, fortified fruit juices, and non-dairy milks

Fiber

You probably think of fiber as something you need for digestion and regular bowel movements, but dietary fiber has many other benefits as well: Diets high in fiber have been linked with reduced risks of cardiovascular disease, type 2 diabetes, and some cancers, as well as a healthier weight. Overall, fiber may be a key contributor to "successful aging," defined as reaching old age free of chronic disease and fully functional.

Australian researchers analyzed data on 1,609 initially healthy people, ages 49 and older, to compare carbohydrate intake and health outcomes. Only 249 participants achieved the goal of "successful aging." The participants who had the highest intake of fiber—an average of 37 grams per day—had an almost 80 percent greater likelihood of living a healthy life during a 10-year follow-up period; they were less likely to suffer from hypertension, diabetes, dementia, depression, and functional disability.

Despite the numerous health benefits of dietary fiber, few Americans meet the recommendations from the DGA: at least 28 grams a day of fiber for men over age 50 and 22 grams for women over age 50, with higher amounts for younger adults. To boost fiber intake, Americans need to increase their consumption of beans and peas, vegetables, fruits, whole grains, and whole-grain products, including cereals, pastas, and breads.

Fiber from Plants

Fiber is found only in plant foods—whole grains, fruits, vegetables, legumes, seeds, and nuts. Refined grains, such as white flour, have been stripped of most of their fiber during processing.

Substituting whole-grain for refined-grain products in your diet will generally increase your fiber intake, although not all whole grains are high in fiber. Whole-wheat bread typically contains 2 grams of fiber per slice—still more than white bread, with 0.8 grams of fiber per slice. A cup of cooked long-grain brown rice has 3.2 grams of fiber, but that's more than five times the fiber (0.6 grams) in white rice (a refined grain). Quinoa has more fiber than most grains, with more than 5 grams per cup of cooked quinoa. Bulgur wheat is richest in fiber, with 8 grams per cup of cooked grains.

At snack time, boost your fiber intake with nuts—just one-quarter cup of walnuts, for example, has 2 grams of fiber.

Choosing Fiber Foods

Eating a variety of plant-based foods will ensure that you're getting enough of both types of fiber: soluble (absorbs water) and insoluble. There's no single "best" way to add fiber to your diet.

An easy way to increase your fiber intake is to substitute fiber-rich choices for foods already in your diet, rather than adding extra foods to boost your fiber intake. If you buy high-fiber processed foods, such as packaged granola bars, be aware that unhealthy added sugars often accompany the healthy fiber.

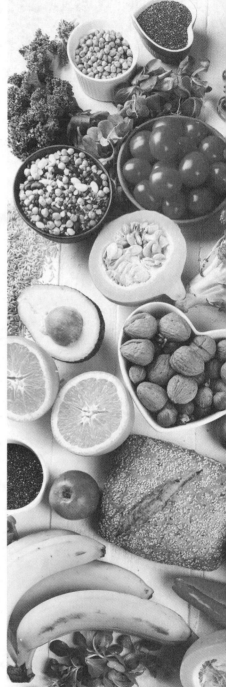

© Tatjana Baibakova | Dreamstime

Good sources of fiber include whole grains, beans, fruits, vegetables, nuts, and seeds.

Foods High in Fiber

FOOD	FIBER CONTENT (GRAMS)
Navy beans, cooked, ½ cup	9.5
100% bran ready-to-eat cereal, ½ cup	8.8
Chia seeds, 2 Tbsp	8.2
Split peas, cooked, ½ cup	8.1
Lentils, cooked, ½ cup	7.5
Black beans, cooked, ½ cup	6.6
Lima beans, cooked, ½ cup	6.5
Chickpeas, cooked, ½ cup	6.2
Shredded wheat ready-to-eat cereal, 1 cup	4.8
Sweet potato, baked, with skin, 1 medium	4.4
Acorn squash, cooked, ½ cup	4.3
Whole-wheat English muffin, 1 regular	4.1
Pear, raw, 1 small	4.0
Bulgur, cooked, ½ cup	4.1
Raspberries, raw, ½ cup	4.0
Apple with skin, 1 medium	3.3
Almonds, 1 oz	3.3

Source: USDA

Sources of Fiber

When choosing high-fiber foods, remember that foods made with grains, such as whole-grain breads, rolls, wraps, cereals, and pasta, as well as the grains themselves, can be good sources of fiber.

▶ **Grains:** Wheat and oat bran, bulgur, whole wheat, barley, popcorn, oats, quinoa, rye, spelt, farro, buckwheat, brown rice

▶ **Vegetables:** Beans (black, kidney, navy, lima, white, pinto), peas, artichokes, broccoli, Brussels sprouts, kale, sweet potatoes, carrots, avocados

▶ **Fruits:** Raspberries, pears (with skin), apples (with skin), blackberries, strawberries, bananas, figs, oranges, mangoes, guava

▶ **Nuts and Seeds:** Pumpkin seeds, chia seeds, flaxseed, sesame seeds, sunflower seeds, pistachios, hazelnuts, almonds, pine nuts, pecans

Vitamin B_{12}

Research has demonstrated a link between vitamin B_{12} levels and brain function. Low levels of vitamin B_{12} have been linked to poorer scores on cognitive tests, including memory tests, and to smaller total brain volume. Even if you're just a little low in vitamin B_{12}, you might be at risk for cognitive decline, according to Tufts researchers. Their analysis of data collected from people with an average age of 75 found that declines in cognitive abilities over an eight-year period were greater in those with the lowest vitamin B_{12} levels than in those with higher B_{12} levels.

Aging and B_{12} Deficiency

Getting enough vitamin B_{12} can be especially challenging for older adults because it often becomes more difficult to absorb B_{12} from food as you age. Older people produce less stomach acid and frequently take acid-reducing medications for heartburn and gastroesophageal reflux disease (GERD), and acid is needed to release vitamin B_{12} from proteins with which it is coupled. And you might be deficient in vitamin B_{12} if you follow a vegetarian or vegan diet, because B_{12} is found only in animal-sourced foods.

Fortunately, the form of vitamin B_{12} in supplements and fortified foods doesn't require an acidic environment for absorption.

Sources of Vitamin B_{12}

▶ **Seafood:** Sardines, salmon, tuna, mackerel, herring, cod, clams, oysters, scallops, mussels, crab

▶ **Dairy:** Milk, yogurt, cheese, eggs

▶ **Fortified foods:** Ready-to-eat breakfast cereals, soymilk and other non-dairy beverages (check the labels for B_{12})

Antioxidants

You've seen the commercials about the "miraculous" power of antioxidants. But before you buy pricey "superfood" beverages or supplements that contain antioxidants, remember that these nutrients can be obtained from the foods and beverages found in healthy dietary patterns.

What exactly are "antioxidants," anyway? They include vitamins C and E, carotenoids such as beta-carotene and lycopene, and the mineral selenium, as well as many different phytochemicals, notably those called polyphenols. Antioxidants are so named because they reduce oxidative stress that occurs when there is an excess of free radicals, unstable molecules formed during the body's normal metabolic processes. Keeping free radicals in check is believed to reduce the damage they can do to cellular DNA, which is believed to contribute to the development of many chronic diseases.

Evidence for Antioxidants

A diet with a high total antioxidant content, especially from fruits and vegetables, has been linked to a reduced risk

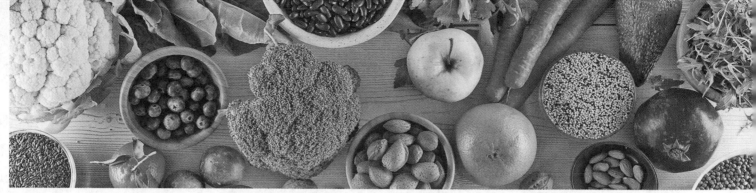

Good sources of antioxidants include brightly colored fruits and vegetables, beans, nuts, seeds, cocoa, and spices.

of stroke, both in people known to have cardiovascular disease and in those initially free of the disease.

Vitamin C appears to protect the endothelium (a layer of cells that lines blood vessels, the heart, and lymph vessels), which may reduce the risk of both heart disease and dementia.

Lycopene, a carotenoid found in tomatoes, watermelon, red bell peppers, and other produce, may reduce your risk of stroke. A study found that men with the highest blood levels of lycopene were 55 percent less likely to suffer a stroke than those with the lowest lycopene levels. Lycopene also may help reduce inflammation and LDL cholesterol, prevent blood clots, and boost immune function.

Vitamin E and Selenium

Diets rich in both vitamin E and the mineral selenium have been linked to a lower risk of age-related cognitive decline. In one study, researchers found that, among adults age 55 and older, those who consumed the most vitamin E from foods were the least likely to develop Alzheimer's disease and other forms of dementia. Another study that measured the selenium levels of elderly people found that those with the highest levels scored 10 years younger on tests of cognitive function compared to those with the lowest levels.

Getting extra vitamin E and selenium, however, may not have extra brain benefits. A long-term study of men who took daily vitamin E and selenium supplements found that neither supplement was linked with a lower risk of dementia. The researchers commented, "For consumers specifically concerned about brain health and cognition, they should be aware that no scientifically rigorous studies have identified any supplement as an effective treatment or prevention for dementia."

The advice to skip supplements is smart for other antioxidants, too. Antioxidants in foods provide the most benefit when they are consumed along with the many other nutrients the foods contain. In many studies, antioxidants in supplement form have failed to show significant protective effects.

Sources of Antioxidant Nutrients

▶ **Beta-carotene:** Sweet potatoes, carrots, spinach, leafy greens, tomatoes, broccoli, winter squash, peaches, mangoes, apricots, cantaloupe, milk, eggs

▶ **Vitamin C:** Kiwifruit, watermelon, oranges, grapefruit, bell peppers, tomatoes, broccoli, strawberries, papaya, pineapple, cabbage, sweet and white potatoes, cantaloupe

▶ **Vitamin E:** Sunflower, safflower and other liquid vegetable oils, almonds and other nuts, sunflower seeds, wheat germ, avocados, shrimp, fortified breakfast cereals

▶ **Lycopene:** Tomatoes and tomato products, grapefruit, watermelon, red bell peppers, guava, papaya, mangos, red cabbage

▶ **Selenium:** Brazil nuts, tuna, sunflower seeds, whole-grain breads and cereals, wheat germ

You don't need to go searching for nutrients that are essential to heart and brain health; you'll find them in a healthy dietary pattern.

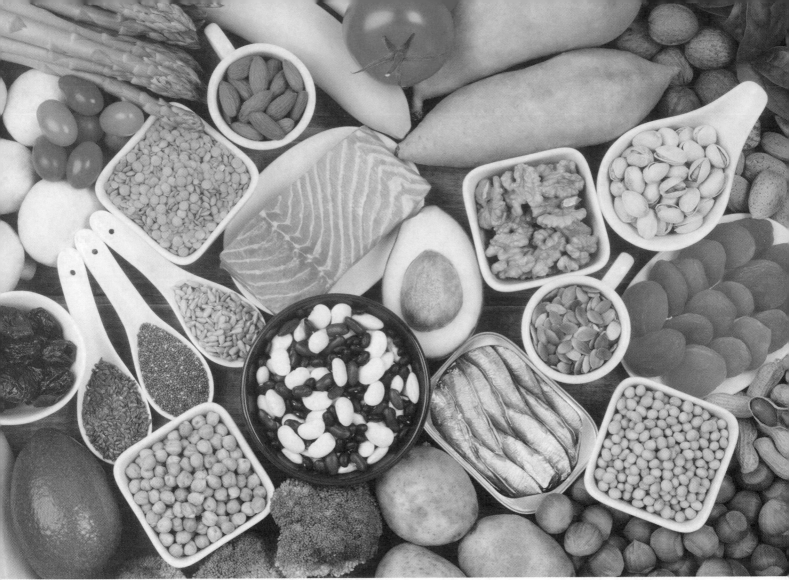

All foods contain one or more of three macronutrients—protein, carbohydrate, and fat.

6 Understanding Macronutrients

Macronutrients—proteins, carbohydrates ("carbs"), and fats—are the three types of nutrients you need in the largest amounts. Your body requires these nutrients for growth, energy, and bodily functions, and they are the sources of calories. (Micronutrients, such as vitamins and minerals, are needed in smaller amounts and are not assigned calorie values.) Food marketers will try to convince you that you need more protein, fewer carbs, or different types of fat—and, often, they say their advice is based on "research." But many claims have not been proven in well-controlled, reliable studies on humans. This chapter will tell you the facts about macronutrients and your heart and brain health.

Protein

You might think that Americans are suffering from a critical shortfall of protein, based on all of the high-protein food and beverage products you see. In fact, most Americans get plenty of protein. The more common problem with protein is the saturated fat, added sugar, and/or high sodium content that may accompany our protein choices.

For example, some high-protein nutrition bars contain five or more teaspoons of added sugar in one 2.5-ounce bar, and an even smaller piece of beef jerky—just 1.25 ounces—may contain 600 or 700 milligrams of sodium, more than 25 percent of your sodium target for the entire day.

Diets such as the so-called Paleo plan, which advocate eating more meat to emulate our ancient ancestors, have little basis in science and only limited evidence for any benefits. For many people, "going paleo" becomes just an excuse for carnivorous indulgence, with predictable waistline results.

Building Blocks

Proteins are found in the cells and tissues of all living things. They are chains of amino acids, molecules that are involved in a variety of biological functions. There are 20 amino acids, nine of which cannot be synthesized in the human body and must be acquired through diet. These are known as essential amino acids. Animal sources of protein (and a select few plant proteins including soy and quinoa) are considered "complete" in that they contain adequate amounts of all the essential amino acids the human body needs.

Your heart needs amino acids to build cardiac muscle. Cardiac muscle is essential for keeping your heart pumping. Other amino acids from proteins make hemoglobin, the component of red blood cells that carries oxygen throughout your body.

Your brain also relies on amino acids for a number of important processes. Amino acids are used in the production and regulation of chemical messengers called neurotransmitters, such as dopamine, norepinephrine, and serotonin, which carry critical information from one nerve cell in the brain to another.

Protein from Plants

Don't be concerned that plant sources of protein are not "complete" proteins. A dietary pattern that includes both whole grains and legumes, for example, will provide a sufficient amount of all nine essential amino acids that must come from dietary sources. Previously, it was thought that complementary foods like these needed to be consumed at the same time, but scientists have proven that eating a variety of plant foods throughout the day can provide all of the amino acids the body needs.

Are you worried that plant proteins will leave you feeling hungry? Research has shown that meals based on plant protein sources like beans are just as filling and satisfying as meals containing animal proteins. For people who choose an entirely plant-based diet, eating a wide variety of plant foods including beans, grains, and nuts will ensure that the body's essential amino acid requirements are met.

Sources of Protein

▶ **Animal sources:** Meat, poultry, seafood, yogurt, milk, cheese, eggs
▶ **Plant sources:** Soybeans and soy products, quinoa, beans, lentils, peas, nuts, seeds, whole grains, meat substitutes

Carbohydrates

Like protein, carbs are the subject of much hype and confusion. Your heart and brain both need carbs, but it's important to get more of the healthy carbs that provide your body with energy that's gradually released, rather than refined carbs (usually, white flour) and added sugars (sugar is a carbohydrate) that will give you a burst of energy but then leave you feeling tired and hungry.

The Nutrition Facts label lists quantities per serving of total carbs, dietary fiber, and sugars. The amount of starch isn't listed, but that's the third component of carbs: Subtract fiber and sugar from the total and the remaining carbs represent starches.

Energy from Glucose

Though it's important not to overdo your intake of sugars and starches, these carbs feed your body in the form of glucose, a simple sugar that is released when carb-containing foods are broken down in your digestive system. For your heart, glucose is the "fuel" that provides the energy to keep pumping.

Your brain also relies on glucose as its primary energy source—and it demands a disproportionately large share. Glucose is among the few substances able to pass unhindered through the blood-brain barrier. Because brain cells can't store glucose, they require a steady stream of glucose throughout the day. Areas of the brain that control thinking are sensitive to drops in glucose, which is why you might have trouble concentrating or thinking clearly if it's been several hours since your last meal.

Carbs for Your Brain

The Recommended Dietary Allowance (RDA) for carbohydrates is actually based on the brain's glucose needs. For adults of all ages, the RDA is 130 grams daily (the equivalent of 520 calories). The Institute of Medicine (IOM) suggests that carbohydrates account for 45 to 65 percent of your total calories; other recommendations vary.

The key to consuming carbohydrates is to ensure that they are good sources of important nutrients. Avoid foods and beverages that are high in carbs from added sugar and/or refined flour, such as soft drinks, white bread, and desserts, which have minimal nutritional value. The *Dietary Guidelines for Americans* stress the importance of limiting carbs in the form of added sugars, as we've already discussed in Chapter 4.

Avoid Starch Surplus

Emerging evidence also suggests that you limit the amount of starches you consume. Research has spotlighted starches as a culprit in weight gain and diabetes, both of which contribute to your risk for cardiovascular disease. One study, for example, reported that high intakes of starchy vegetables such as corn, peas, and potatoes were associated with weight gain. In the same study, diets higher in fruits and non-starchy vegetables were linked with weight loss.

Potatoes were the number-one culprit in weight gain among study participants. "It didn't matter whether they were boiled or baked or mashed or French fries or had fat in them or didn't have fat in them. It was the starch," says Tufts' Dariush Mozaffarian, MD, DrPH, senior author of the study. The weight gain associated with starches from refined grains was identical to that from sugar-sweetened foods.

A simple rule of thumb, Dr. Mozaffarian says, is to look for foods with a ratio of total carbohydrates to fiber of 10:1 or less. For example, a product such as white bread with 15 grams of carbohydrates and one gram of fiber would have a ratio of 15:1—not a good choice. Foods with the recommended ratio of 10:1 or less include all types of beans, peas, and lentils, many whole grains and whole-grain products, and most fruits and vegetables.

Sources of Healthy Carbohydrates

- **Fruits and vegetables:** Beans, lentils, peas, sweet potatoes, apples, pears, berries, bananas, grapes, prunes, figs, dates, melon, broccoli, Brussels sprouts, cauliflower, artichokes
- **Grains:** Whole grains (whole wheat, oats, quinoa, barley, bulgur wheat, popcorn) and most breads, pasta, and cereals made from these whole grains
- **Dairy:** Milk, yogurt, and cheeses, including cottage cheese

Fats

The third macronutrient is fat. We've already seen how it's important to limit saturated fats, and that some plant foods are good sources of unsaturated fat.

Does substituting unsaturated fats for saturated fats really make a difference? A large study reported an 18 percent increased risk of heart disease associated with the highest intake of the most commonly consumed types of saturated fat. The study also showed that replacing saturated fat with polyunsaturated fat (such as in liquid vegetable oils, nuts, and seafood) was associated with lower heart disease risk.

Omega Fatty Acids

Another benefit of substituting unsaturated fats for saturated fats is that these healthy fats include the only types of fat your body can't make on its own: omega-3 and omega-6 fatty acids. Both are subclasses of polyunsaturated fatty acids. You must obtain these "essential" fatty acids from your diet.

When your body digests fats, it breaks them down into fatty acid molecules. The membranes that make up neurons—the brain cells that communicate with one another—are made up of these fatty acids. Fats (along with amino acids) also are used to create myelin, the protective sheath that covers neurons.

Omega-3 Fatty Acids. Fatty acids found in fish oil and in some plants seem to have benefits for both your heart and your brain. Omega-3 fatty acids include alpha-linolenic acid (ALA), found in plants, and eicosapentaenoic acid (EPA) and docosahexaenoic acid (DHA), which are found in fatty fish. The "omega-3" name refers to their molecular structure.

The body converts a small portion of ALA to brain-active, heart-healthy DHA and EPA. Fish and shellfish are the best sources of EPA and DHA. The American Heart Association recommends eating fish (particularly fatty fish) at least two times a week.

Fatty fish such as salmon, mackerel, herring, lake trout, sardines, and albacore tuna are high in EPA and DHA. If you don't care for these fish, don't worry; many other varieties of seafood, including whitefish (tilapia, cod, pollock, flounder, snapper, mahi mahi, swordfish, bass)

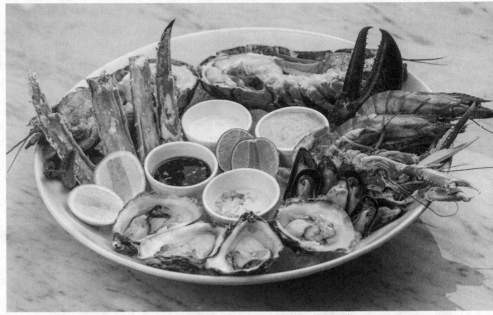
© Artur Begel | Dreamstime

Shellfish provide moderate amounts of omega-3 fatty acids.

and shellfish (oysters, mussels, clams, crab, lobster, shrimp, and scallops) provide smaller amounts of omega-3s.

Research has shown that omega-3 fatty acids like those in fish decrease the risk of arrhythmias (erratic heartbeat), which can lead to strokes. Omega-3s also decrease triglyceride levels, slow the growth of atherosclerotic plaque, and slightly lower blood pressure.

All of the types of omega-3s (ALA, DHA, and EPA) have beneficial effects on cholesterol levels. One study reported that people who consumed 1.5 ounces of walnuts (rich in ALA) six days per week reduced their total cholesterol and LDL ("bad") cholesterol, and those who ate fish twice a week had an increase in HDL ("good") cholesterol and a decrease in triglycerides.

Omega-3 Brain Benefits. The omega-3 DHA is the most plentiful fatty acid in the brain, especially in the neurons and the gray matter—the area responsible for language, memory, and thought. DHA is essential for the proper growth and function of brain tissue, including the production of neurons and the transmission of nerve impulses across neurons. High blood levels of DHA have been linked to a reduced risk of dementia and Alzheimer's disease. Total polyunsaturated fat intake (including omega-3s) has also been inversely linked to the risk of mild cognitive impairment.

A review of 21 observational studies assessed intake of fish and their polyunsaturated fats along with cognitive changes in middle-aged and older adults for up to two decades. Researchers found that eating one additional serving per week of fish was associated with a 7 percent lower risk of Alzheimer's disease, compared to not eating fish. Eating an extra weekly serving of fish was associated with a 5 percent overall lower risk of dementia. Each daily increment of 8 grams of polyunsaturated fats was associated with a 29 percent lower risk of mild cognitive impairment and a 10 percent lower risk of Parkinson's disease.

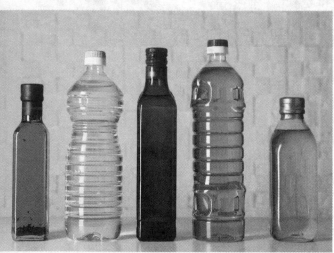

© Chernetskaya | Dreamstime

Vegetable oils are good sources of linoleic acid, an essential omega-6 fatty acid.

Omega-6 Fatty Acids. Less talked about in the news than omega-3s, omega-6 fatty acids are nonetheless common. Linoleic acid (LA) is the essential omega-6 fatty acid that is most plentiful in vegetable oils, nuts, and seeds. Linoleic acid is necessary for normal growth, development, and brain function.

Swapping sources of omega-6 fatty acids for foods high in saturated fat has cardiovascular benefits. One study found that substituting 5 percent of calories consumed from saturated fat with foods containing linoleic acid was associated with a 9 percent lower risk of coronary heart disease events and a 13 percent lower coronary heart disease mortality risk. Substituting linoleic acid for 5 percent of calories from carbohydrates was also associated with reductions in risks associated with heart disease.

Some experts have recommended lowering the intake of omega-6 fats, arguing that omega-6s might be linked to inflammation. An American Heart Association review, however, indicated that the consumption of at least 5 percent to 10 percent of energy from omega-6s reduces the risk of heart disease. It suggested that higher intakes of omega-6s "appear to be safe and may be even more beneficial (as part of a low–saturated-fat, low-cholesterol diet)."

Omega-9 Fatty Acids. Unlike omega-3s and omega-6s, the body can produce omega-9 fatty acids, so these are not considered "essential." Because these are also unsaturated fats, however, they are also a healthy substitute for saturated fats. The main omega-9 is oleic acid, a monounsaturated fat found in vegetable oils, avocados, and many other foods.

Sources of Healthy Fats

▶ **ALA:** Flaxseed, walnuts, other nuts and seeds, wheat germ, soy foods

▶ **DHA and EPA:** Salmon, sardines, mackerel, trout, tuna, swordfish, bass, carp, flounder, tilapia, oysters, clams, scallops, shrimp

▶ **Linoleic acid:** Liquid vegetable oils (sunflower, safflower, soybean, canola, grapeseed, olive, corn, peanut), nuts and seeds

▶ **Oleic acid:** Vegetable and nut oils (olive, sunflower, canola, peanut, macadamia), avocados, nuts and seeds

With the macronutrients, we've finished exploring the basics of a dietary pattern that supports heart and brain health, as well as the foods and nutrients that are the key ingredients in that pattern. Now it's time to show you how to put this information into practice with heart-brain healthy recipes and recommendations for breakfast, lunch, dinner, and even snacks and desserts.

7 2020 Heart-Brain Diet Recipes

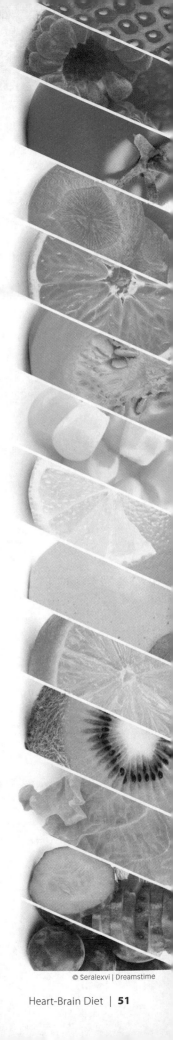

BREAKFAST

LUNCH

SNACK

DINNER

DESSERT

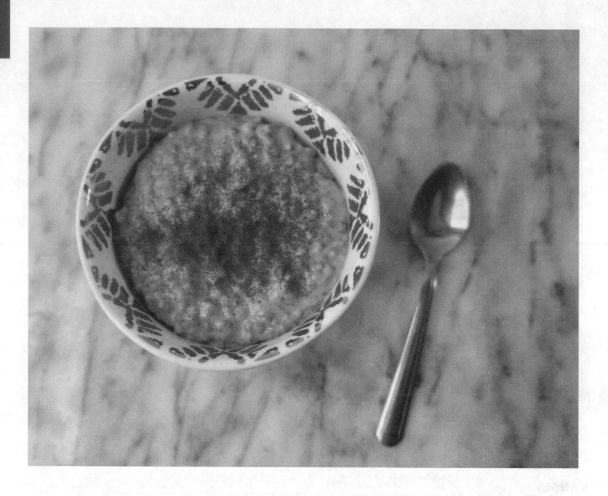

Apricot and Tahini Steel-Cut Oats

Ingredients

1½ cups milk

½ cup steel-cut oats, uncooked

2 apricots, diced

1 Tbsp tahini

1 tsp honey

Cinnamon, to taste

Steps

1. In a small, heavy-bottomed saucepan over medium-high heat, heat milk and oats, stirring occasionally, until tiny bubbles just begin to form around the sides of the pan. Add apricots, tahini, and honey to pan; stir to combine.
2. Reduce heat to medium-low, cover, and simmer for 15-20 minutes, stirring occasionally.
3. Remove from heat and let stand covered for 5 minutes. Divide oatmeal into two bowls; top each bowl with a sprinkle of cinnamon.

Yield: 2 servings

Per serving: 290 calories, 7 g total fat, 1 g sat fat, 13 g protein, 45 g carbs, 5g fiber, 16 g sugar, 80 mg sodium

Recipe (adapted) and photo: Oldways, www.oldwayspt.org

Pumpkin-Granola Parfait

Ingredients

1 (15 oz) can low-sodium pumpkin

3 cups fat-free or low-fat vanilla yogurt

¼ tsp ground cinnamon

¼ tsp ground nutmeg

½ cup quick-cooking oats

½ cup rice crisps

¼ cup raisins

1 Tbsp vegetable oil

¼ cup brown (or white) sugar

Steps

1. Preheat oven to 325°F.
2. In a blender or with a fork, blend the pumpkin until smooth.
3. Mix pumpkin, yogurt, and spices in a bowl.
4. In another bowl, mix together the oats, rice crisps, raisins, oil, and sugar. Spread the oat mixture (granola) on a baking pan; bake for 10 minutes. Let the granola cool down until it hardens. Then, break it apart or crush it into small pieces.
5. Spoon about ¼ cup of the pumpkin mixture into 6 medium-size glasses. Sprinkle about 2 tablespoons of granola on top of the pumpkin mixture in each glass.
6. Continue to alternate the pumpkin mixture and granola in layers, ending with granola. Serve immediately or refrigerate.

Yield: 6 (1-cup) servings

Per serving: 226 calories, 5 g total fat, 1 g sat fat, 8 g protein, 40 g carbs, 3 g fiber, 29 g sugar, 107 mg sodium

Recipe (adapted) and photo: USDA Harvest of Healthy Recipes

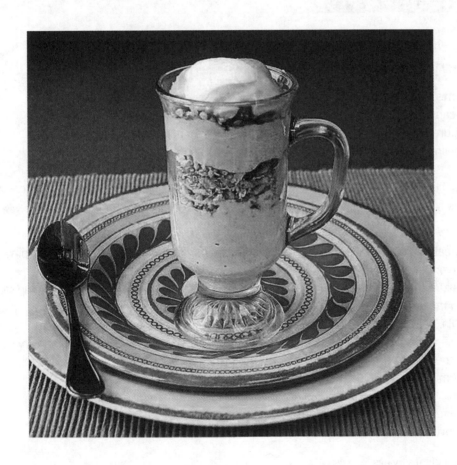

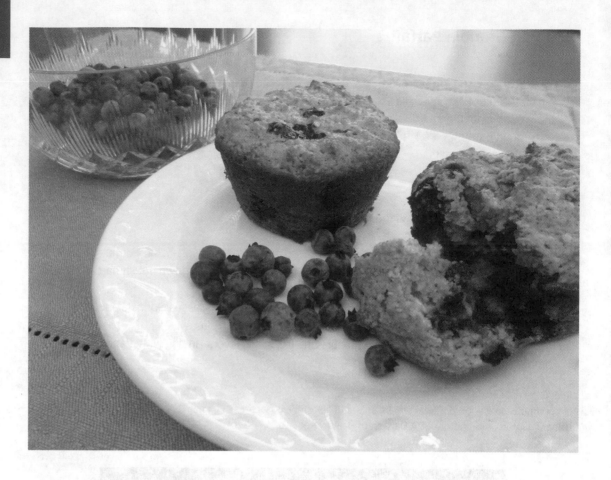

Blueberry Whole-Grain Muffins

Ingredients

3 Tbsp canola oil

½ cup pure maple syrup

1 cup plain low-fat yogurt

1 egg

1 tsp vanilla extract

1⅓ cups whole-wheat pastry flour

1 cup rolled oats

2 tsp baking powder

¾ tsp salt

½ tsp cinnamon

¼ tsp baking soda

1 cup fresh blueberries

Steps

1. Preheat oven to 400°F. Prepare a 12-cup standard muffin tin with nonstick cooking spray and flour, or paper baking cups.
2. Measure the oil into a 1-cup measuring cup; add the maple syrup to the oil. (The syrup slips easily from the measuring cup due to the oil.) Pour oil and syrup into a large bowl; add yogurt, egg, and vanilla. Beat vigorously with a spoon or whisk until ingredients are well mixed.
3. In a separate bowl, stir together all dry ingredients except the blueberries. Add the dry ingredients and the blueberries to the wet ingredients and stir until just combined. Do not overmix (overmixing will produce dense, rubbery muffins).
4. Spoon the batter into the muffin tin, filling each cup just short of the top.
5. Bake for 18-20 minutes, until tops are browned and a toothpick comes out clean.
6. Remove from oven and cool for 10 minutes before removing to a cooling rack.

Yield: 12 (1 muffin) servings

Per serving: 157 calories, 5 g total fat, 1 g sat fat, 5 g protein, 28 g carbs, 3 g fiber, 11 g sugar, 277 mg sodium

Recipe (adapted) and photo: Oldways, www.oldwayspt.org

Breakfast Burrito with Salsa

Ingredients

4 large eggs

2 Tbsp frozen corn

1 Tbsp 1% milk

2 Tbsp diced red or green pepper

¼ cup minced onion

1 clove garlic, minced

1 Tbsp diced fresh tomatoes

1 tsp mustard*

¼ tsp hot pepper sauce (optional)

4 (8-inch) whole-wheat flour tortillas

½ cup prepared salsa**

Steps

1. Preheat oven to 350°F.
2. In a large mixing bowl, blend the eggs, corn, milk, green peppers, onions, tomatoes, mustard, garlic, hot pepper sauce, and salt for 1 minute until eggs are smooth.
3. Pour egg mixture into a lightly oiled 9"x9" baking dish and cover with foil.
4. Bake for 20-25 minutes until eggs are set and thoroughly cooked.
5. Place tortillas on microwave-safe plate, cover with paper towel, and microwave for 10-20 seconds until warm.
6. Cut baked egg mixture into 4 equal pieces; roll 1 piece of cooked egg in each tortilla.
7. Serve each burrito topped with 2 Tbsp of salsa.

    * May use brown or Dijon mustard in place of yellow mustard.

    ** To reduce sodium content, choose low-sodium or no-salt-added salsa.

Yield: 4 servings

Per serving: 233 calories, 9 g total fat, 3 g sat fat, 11 g protein, 29 g carbs, 4 g fiber, 3 g sugar, 491 mg sodium

Recipe (adapted): USDA Healthy Eating on a Budget

Photo: © Svetlana Foote | Dreamstime

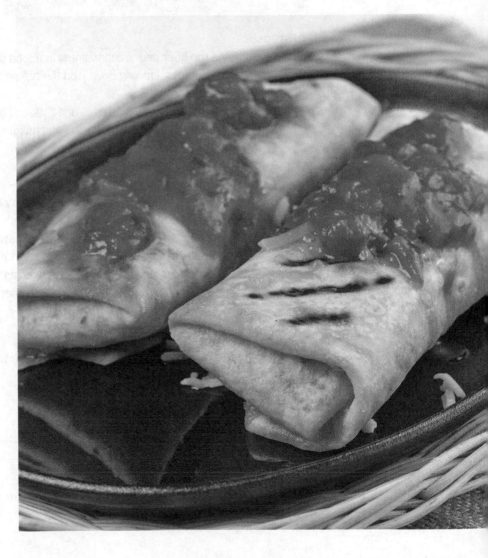

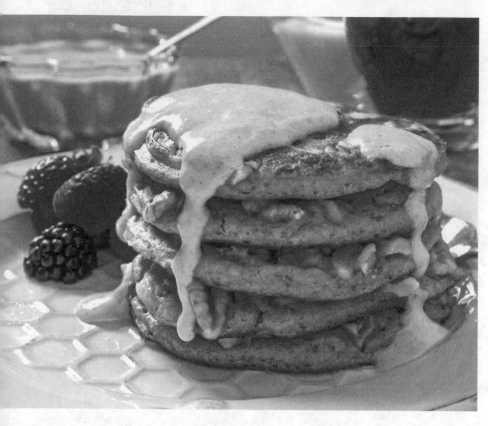

Whole-Wheat Walnut Pancakes

Ingredients

Pancakes:
1 cup whole-wheat flour
⅔ cup finely chopped walnuts
1 Tbsp baking powder
¼ tsp baking soda
¼ tsp salt
2 eggs
1 cup plus 2 Tbsp milk (and additional
    milk if needed)
2 Tbsp unsweetened applesauce
1 Tbsp maple syrup

Pumpkin yogurt sauce:
1¼ cups plain nonfat yogurt
    (without stabilizers)
½ cup cooked, mashed pumpkin or
    canned pumpkin
⅓ cup apple cider
1 Tbsp maple syrup
2 tsp pumpkin pie spice

Steps

1. Combine the flour and ⅓ cup walnuts in a food processor and pulse until the walnuts are finely ground. Pour into a mixing bowl; add the baking powder, baking soda, and salt, and stir to combine.

2. In a separate bowl, combine eggs and milk and beat until blended. Add the applesauce and maple syrup and stir until smooth. Pour the egg mixture over the flour mixture and stir just until the dry ingredients are moistened.

3. Combine all sauce ingredients in a medium saucepan and whisk until smooth. Before serving, warm gently over low heat, stirring frequently–don't let it boil.

4. Spray a large nonstick skillet with cooking spray and place over medium-high heat. When the skillet is hot, spoon the batter onto it, using about 3 tablespoons of batter for each pancake; a 12-inch skillet will hold four pancakes. (If the batter seems too thick, add another 1-2 tablespoons of milk.) Sprinkle each pancake with about 1 teaspoon of the remaining chopped walnuts. Cook until the pancakes look dry around the edges and bubbles break on the surface, about 2 minutes. Turn and cook about 1 minute more on the other side. Serve the pancakes hot, with pumpkin yogurt sauce.

YIELD: 7 servings (2 pancakes)
Per serving: 242 calories, 12 g total fat, 2 g sat fat, 10 g protein, 24 g carbs, 3 g fiber, 12 g sugar, 349 mg sodium
Recipe (adapted) and photo: California Walnuts

Pita Pizzas

Ingredients

1 cup Super-Quick Chunky Tomato Sauce (see recipe below); low-sodium tomato-based pasta sauce may be substituted

1 cup cooked boneless, skinless chicken breast, diced

1 cup cooked broccoli, chopped

2 Tbsp grated Parmesan cheese

1 Tbsp fresh basil, chopped (or 1 tsp dried)

4 (6½-inch) whole-wheat pitas

Steps

1. Preheat oven or toaster oven to 450°F.
2. For each pizza, spread ¼ cup tomato sauce on a pita and top with ¼ cup chicken, ¼ cup broccoli, ½ tablespoon Parmesan cheese, and ¼ tablespoon chopped basil.
3. Place pitas on a nonstick baking sheet and bake for about 5–8 minutes until golden brown and chicken is heated through. Serve immediately.

Yield: 4 servings (1 pita each, with sauce)

Per serving: 248 calories, 5 g total fat, 1 g sat fat, 19 g protein, 37 g carbs, 6 g fiber, 3 g sugar, 597 mg sodium

Recipe (adapted) and photo: National Heart, Lung & Blood Institute, wecan.nhlbi.nih.gov

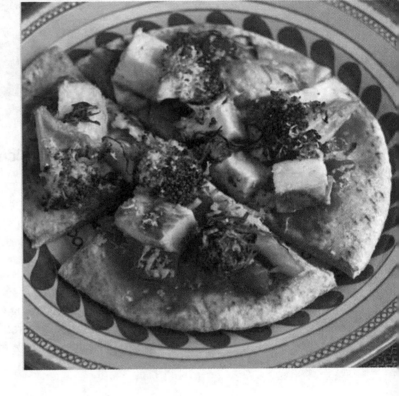

Super-Quick Chunky Tomato Sauce

Ingredients

2 tsp extra-virgin olive oil

1 clove garlic, chopped

1 (12 oz) jar roasted red peppers, drained and diced (or substitute fresh roasted red peppers)

2 (14½ oz) cans no-salt-added diced tomatoes

1 (5½ oz) can low-sodium tomato juice

1 Tbsp fresh basil, chopped (or 1 teaspoon dried)

¼ tsp ground black pepper

Steps

1. In a medium saucepan, heat olive oil over medium heat. Add garlic and cook for 30 seconds, stirring constantly.
2. Add diced red peppers; continue to cook for 2–3 minutes, until the peppers begin to sizzle.
3. Add tomatoes, tomato juice, basil, and pepper. Bring to a boil; reduce heat, and simmer for 10 minutes, or until the sauce thickens slightly.
4. Use immediately or refrigerate in a tightly sealed container for 3–5 days.

Yield: 12 (½-cup) servings

Per serving: 25 calories, 1 g total fat, 0 g sat fat, 1 g protein, 4 g carbs, 2 g fiber, 2 g sugar, 396 mg sodium

Recipe (adapted): National Heart, Lung & Blood Institute, wecan.nhlbi.nih.gov

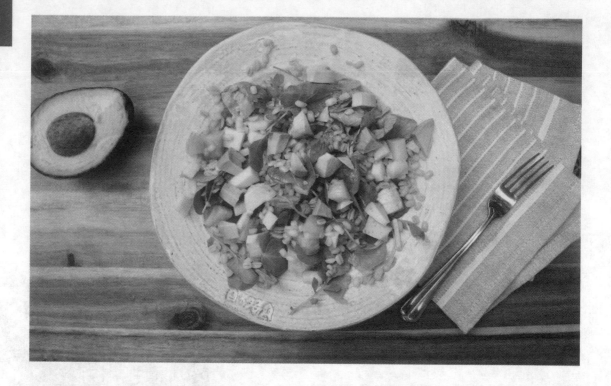

Barley, Pineapple, and Jicama Salad with Avocado

Ingredients
- 1 cup hulled (not pearled or flaked) barley
- 2 Tbsp fresh lime juice
- ¼ cup olive oil
- ¼ tsp ground cumin
- ¼ tsp salt
- ¼ tsp ground black pepper
- 6 cups watercress or 6 cups arugula, washed
- 1 medium jicama, peeled and grated
- 2 cups cubed pineapple (about ½ medium pineapple, peeled and cored)
- 2 large avocados, cubed

Steps
1. Bring barley and 3 cups water to a boil; reduce heat and simmer, covered, for 45-60 minutes, until liquid is absorbed and the grains are tender.
2. While barley is cooking, whisk together lime juice, olive oil, cumin, salt, and pepper.
3. In a large bowl, toss watercress or arugula with half of the dressing.
4. When barley is done cooking, drain off any excess liquid. Add barley, jicama, pineapple, and avocado to the greens along with the rest of the dressing; toss gently to combine.

Yield: 6 servings
Per serving: 349 calories, 17 g total fat, 2 g sat fat, 6 g protein, 48 g carbs, 15 g fiber, 8 g sugar, 116 mg sodium
Recipe (adapted) and photo: Oldways, www.oldwayspt.org

White Chili

- 1 Tbsp extra-virgin olive oil
- 2 red peppers, chopped
- 1 large onion, chopped
- 1 (4 oz) can chopped green chiles (adjust to taste)
- 3 garlic cloves, minced
- 1 Tbsp chili powder
- 1 tsp cumin
- 1 tsp oregano
- 2 cups low-sodium chicken broth
- 2 cups low-fat (1%) milk
- 4 cups low-sodium or no-salt-added canned white beans, drained and rinsed
- 12 oz (about 3 cups) cooked chicken (such as rotisserie chicken), cubed
- 6 (5-inch) corn tortillas, toasted and cut into 1-inch squares
- ¼ cup cilantro (optional)

Steps

1. In a large soup pot or Dutch oven, heat olive oil over medium heat; add peppers and onion and sauté until softened, about 5-7 minutes.
2. Add green chiles, garlic, spices, and chicken broth to pot. Simmer for 20 minutes.
3. Add milk, beans, and cooked chicken to pot; stir to combine. Heat through over medium-low heat.
4. Top chili with cilantro (if using) and crisp tortillas before serving.

Yield: 10 servings
Per serving: 250 calories, 5 g total fat, 1 g sat fat, 22 g protein, 31 g carbs, 7 g fiber, 5 g sugar, 401 mg sodium
Recipe (adapted): USDA Healthy Eating on a Budget
Photo: © Michelle Arnold | Dreamstime

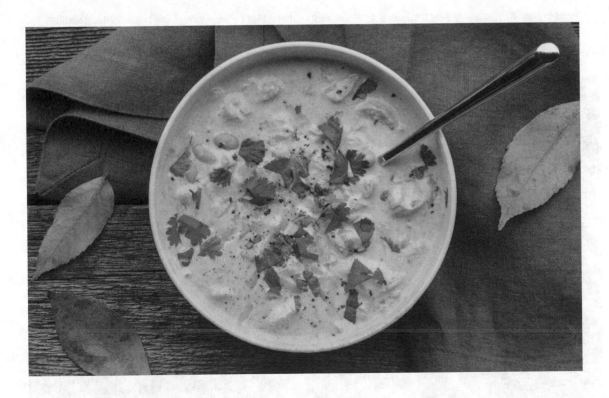

Grilled Chicken Taco Salad

Ingredients

⅓ cup vegetable oil

3 Tbsp freshly squeezed lime juice

1 Tbsp taco seasoning

1¼ lb (20 oz) skinless, boneless chicken breasts, flattened slightly

6 cups romaine lettuce, torn in bite-size pieces

1 cup grape tomatoes, quartered

¼ cup reduced-fat shredded cheddar cheese

1 avocado, peeled and cut into chunks

2 Tbsp sliced black olives

½ cup reduced-fat sour cream

Steps

1. In a 1-cup glass measure, combine the vegetable oil, lime juice, and taco seasoning; mix well. Place the chicken in a medium bowl; pour the marinade on top of the chicken, making sure all surfaces are coated. Refrigerate for 1-2 hours.

2. Prepare a grill or grill pan. Cook the chicken over medium heat for about 6 minutes; turn the chicken over and continue grilling until cooked through (4 to 6 additional minutes). Remove the chicken from the grill. Cut each piece into ¼–inch slices.

3. On 4 individual dinner plates, arrange about 1 cup of lettuce leaves and ¼ cup of tomatoes. Arrange ¼ of chicken strips on the lettuce. Sprinkle each salad with 1 tablespoon cheddar cheese, ¼ of the avocado chunks, and ¼ of the black olives. Top each salad with 2 tablespoons sour cream.

Yield: 4 servings

Per serving: 529 calories, 37 g total fat, 6 g sat fat, 38 g protein, 11 g carbs, 5 g fiber, 3 g sugar, 398 mg sodium

Recipe (adapted) and photo: Daisy Brands

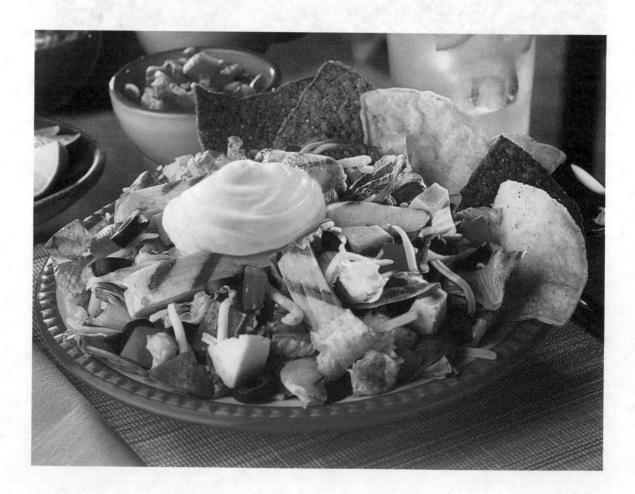

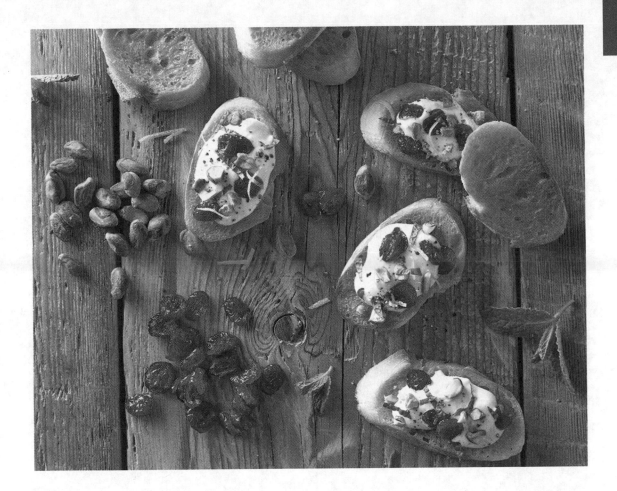

Cranberry Pistachio Crostini

Ingredients

2 Tbsp extra-virgin olive oil

1 baguette or loaf of crusty bread, cut into 10 ¾-inch slices

½ cup low-fat cottage cheese

½ cup reduced-fat sour cream

1 Tbsp grated fresh lemon peel

1½ Tbsp chopped fresh basil

½ Tbsp chopped fresh mint

⅓ cup dried cranberries

⅓ cup coarsely chopped pistachios, roasted, unsalted

⅛ tsp salt

⅛ tsp freshly ground black pepper

Steps

1. Heat oven to 425°F. Line a baking sheet with parchment paper. Brush the olive oil on both sides of the baguette slices and place on baking sheet. Bake for 10-12 minutes or until lightly browned, turning once.

2. Meanwhile, pulse cottage cheese and sour cream in a food processor until smooth. Stir in lemon peel, basil, and mint. Cover and refrigerate until ready to serve.

3. Top toasted bread with cottage cheese mixture. Sprinkle with cranberries and pistachios. Lightly sprinkle with sea salt and pepper. Garnish with mint sprigs and, if desired, very lightly drizzle with extra-virgin olive oil.

Yield: 10 servings

Per serving: 122 calories, 7 g total fat, 2 g sat fat, 4 g protein, 13 g carbs, 1 g fiber, 5 g sugar, 149 mg sodium

Recipe (adapted) and photo: Daisy Brands

Peanut Butter Hummus and Pita Chips

Ingredients

Hummus:

2 cups low-sodium garbanzo beans (chickpeas), rinsed

¼ cup low-sodium chicken broth

¼ cup lemon juice

2-3 Tbsp garlic, diced (about 4–6 garlic cloves, depending on taste)

¼ cup creamy peanut butter (or substitute other nut or seed butter)

¼ tsp cayenne pepper (or substitute paprika for less spice)

1 Tbsp olive oil

Pita chips:

4 (6½-inch) whole-wheat pitas, each cut into 10 triangles

1 Tbsp extra-virgin olive oil

1 tsp (about 1 clove) garlic, minced, or ½ tsp garlic powder

¼ tsp ground black pepper

Steps

1. Preheat oven to 400°F.
2. Place all hummus ingredients in a food processor or blender. Purée until smooth.
3. In a large bowl, toss the pita triangles with the olive oil, garlic, and pepper.
4. Bake pita chips on a baking sheet for 10 minutes or until crispy; serve with hummus.

Yield: 8 servings (⅓ cup hummus and 5 chips)

Per serving: 217 calories, 9 g total fat, 1 g sat fat, 8 g protein, 29 g carbs, 5 g fiber, 4 g sugar, 190 mg sodium

Recipe (Adapted): National Heart, Lung & Blood Institute

Photo: © Scott Karcich | Dreamstime

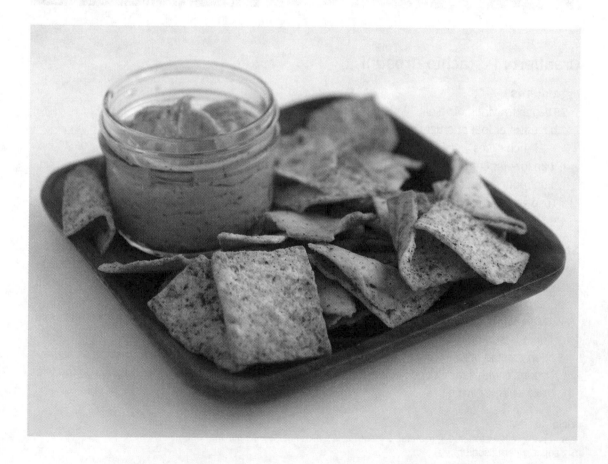

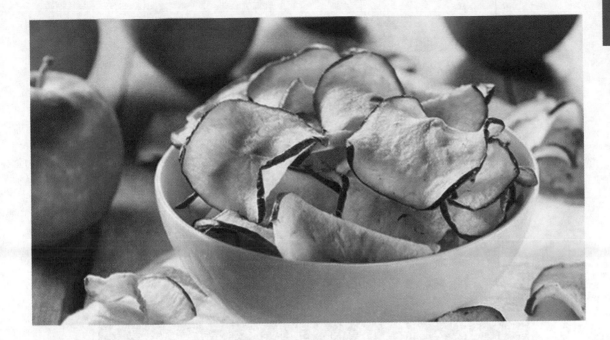

Baked Apple Chips

Ingredients:
- 4 large apples (any variety, unpeeled)
- 2 tsp cinnamon
- 1 Tbsp granulated sugar

Steps
1. Slice apples horizontally into very thin rounds, using a sharp knife or mandolin. Remove any seeds that do not fall out as you cut.
2. Combine cinnamon and sugar.
3. Lay the apple slices in a single layer on a baking sheet lined with parchment paper; sprinkle lightly with the cinnamon sugar.
4. Bake apple slices at 250°F for 1 hour, flip slices, and bake for an additional hour (2 hours total). Chips will continue to crisp up as they cool.

Yield: 8 servings
Per serving: 66 calories, 0 g total fat, 0 g sat fat, 0 g protein, 17 g carbs, 3 g fiber, 13 g sugar, 0 mg sodium
Recipe (adapted) and photo: American Institute for Cancer Research, www.aicr.org

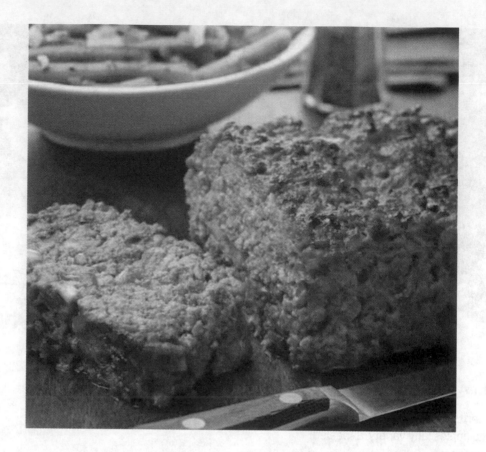

Scrumptious Meat Loaf

Ingredients

1 lb ground beef, 97% lean

½ cup tomato paste

¼ cup onion, chopped

¼ cup green bell pepper, diced

¼ cup red bell pepper, diced

1 cup fresh tomatoes, blanched, chopped

½ tsp low-sodium mustard

¼ tsp ground black pepper

½ tsp hot pepper, chopped (optional)

2 cloves garlic, chopped

2 scallions, chopped

½ tsp ground ginger

⅛ tsp ground nutmeg

1 tsp grated orange rind

½ tsp fresh thyme, crushed, or ⅛ tsp dried thyme

¼ cup fine breadcrumbs

Steps

1. Preheat oven to 350°F.
2. Mix all ingredients together in a large bowl.
3. Place in 1-pound loaf pan (preferably with drip rack) and bake, covered, for 50 minutes.
4. Uncover pan and continue baking for 12 minutes.

Yield: 6 servings (one 1¼-inch-thick slice each)

Per serving: 152 calories, 3 g total fat, 1 g sat fat, 17 g protein, 14 g carbs, 2 g fiber, 5 g sugar, 117 mg sodium

Recipe (adapted) and photo: National Heart, Lung & Blood Institute, wecan.nhlbi.nih.gov

Spinach Pasta Chickpea Salad with Salmon

Ingredients

6 oz whole-grain pasta, uncooked

2 cloves garlic, minced

Juice of 1 lemon

4 Tbsp extra-virgin olive oil

1 (15 oz) can low-sodium chickpeas, rinsed and drained

6 cups chopped spinach leaves, packed

½ cup feta cheese, crumbled

1 lb salmon, fresh or frozen and thawed

Steps

1. Bring a large pot of water to a boil; cook pasta according to instructions (about 8 minutes).
2. While the pasta is cooking combine the garlic, lemon juice, and olive oil in a large bowl.
3. Drain the pasta, allow to cool for a few minutes, and add to bowl. Add spinach leaves and feta; stir to combine.
4. Grill salmon on an outdoor grill or indoor grill pan or under a broiler until fish flakes easily. Time will vary according to thickness of fish but will usually be 10 minutes or less.
5. Divide pasta salad among four plates and top with one-quarter of the cooked salmon. Salad can be served slightly warm or cooled for up to four hours (more may wilt spinach) until you're ready to eat.

Yield: 4 servings

Per serving: 655 calories, 33 g total fat, 7 g sat fat, 38 g protein, 53 g carbs, 10 g fiber, 5 g sugar, 288 mg sodium

Recipe (adapted) and photo: Oldways, www.oldwayspt.org

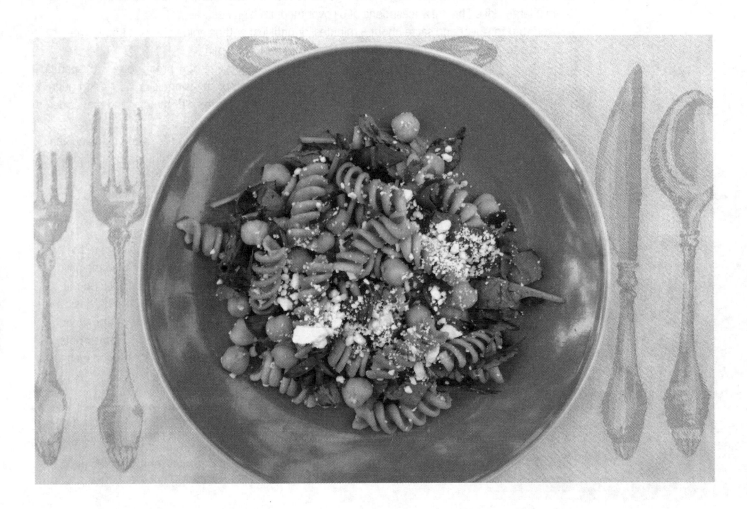

Veggie Pad Thai

Ingredients

Sauce:
1 Tbsp fish sauce

2 Tbsp rice vinegar

1 Tbsp reduced-sodium soy sauce or tamari

1 Tbsp honey

¼ cup lime juice (juice of 1-2 limes)

Pad Thai:
8 oz wide, flat rice noodles
(preferably brown rice noodles), uncooked

1 Tbsp olive, sesame, or canola oil, divided

8 oz extra-firm tofu, drained and cut into
½-inch cubes

2 large eggs

½ yellow onion, chopped

3 cloves garlic, minced

1 head of broccoli, cut into small florets

1 zucchini, spiralized (or sliced into thin,
long strips)

1 cup snap peas

2 carrots, grated

1 cup mung bean sprouts

¼ cup fresh basil, chopped

¼ cup fresh cilantro, chopped

Crushed red pepper, to taste

Garnishes:
2 Tbsp peanuts, chopped

Lime wedges

Steps

1. In a small bowl, whisk together all the sauce ingredients; set aside.
2. Prepare the noodles according to package instructions. Drain noodles and set aside.
3. In a large skillet, heat 1½ teaspoons of oil over medium-high heat.
4. Add tofu to skillet and sauté about 3 minutes, or until just getting golden brown. Rotate the pieces to get a golden color on all sides. Move tofu to edge of pan.

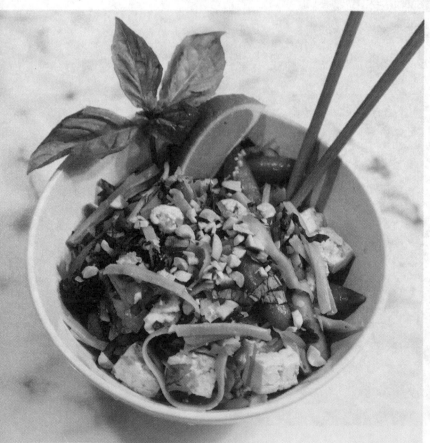

5. Crack eggs into pan, break yolks with spatula, and scramble eggs until just cooked through (about 1 minute). Set the egg and tofu aside on a plate.
6. Add remaining oil to pan. Add onion and garlic to pan and sauté 1-2 minutes, or until just translucent.
7. Add broccoli, zucchini, snap peas, and carrots; sauté until they are just fork-tender and still bright in color, about 3 minutes.
8. Add noodles, sauce, tofu, and eggs to the pan. Gently mix everything together so the flavors combine and the noodles can soak up the sauce. Add half of the bean sprouts, basil, and cilantro, mix gently, and remove from heat.
9. Serve topped with remaining bean sprouts, basil, and cilantro, peanuts, and lime wedges on the side.

Yield: 4 servings (1 ½-2 cups each)

Per serving: 475 calories, 13 g total fat, 2 g sat fat, 21 g protein, 74 g carbs, 9 g fiber, 13 g sugar, 647 mg sodium

Recipe (adapted) and photo: American Institute for Cancer Research, www.aicr.org

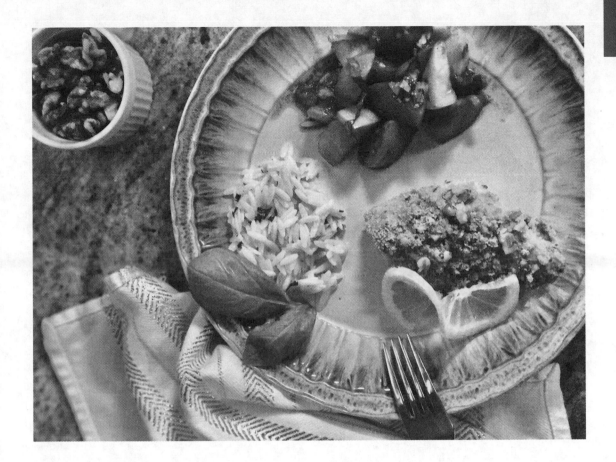

Walnut-Encrusted Tilapia

Ingredients

1 Tbsp extra-virgin olive oil, divided

1 large egg

Zest of 1 lemon

1 clove garlic, finely chopped

1 Tbsp grated Parmesan cheese

⅛ tsp salt

Pepper to taste

¼ cup finely chopped walnuts

⅔ cup whole-wheat breadcrumbs

1 lb tilapia, fresh or frozen and thawed

Steps

1. Preheat oven to 425°F. Coat 9" x 13" baking dish with 1 tsp olive oil.
2. Beat egg in mixing bowl; add lemon zest, remaining olive oil, garlic, Parmesan cheese, salt, and pepper, and whisk together.
3. Mix walnuts and breadcrumbs together in a pie pan or large, shallow bowl.
4. Dip fish into egg mixture. Dredge in breadcrumb mixture, coating both sides well. Place breaded fillets in prepared baking dish.
5. Bake for 17 minutes or until fillets appear opaque and fish flakes easily with a fork.

Yield: 4 servings

Per serving: 282 calories, 13 g total fat, 2 g sat fat, 29 g protein, 15 g carbs, 3 g fiber, 1 g sugar, 190 mg sodium

Recipe (adapted) and photo: American Institute for Cancer Research, www.aicr.org

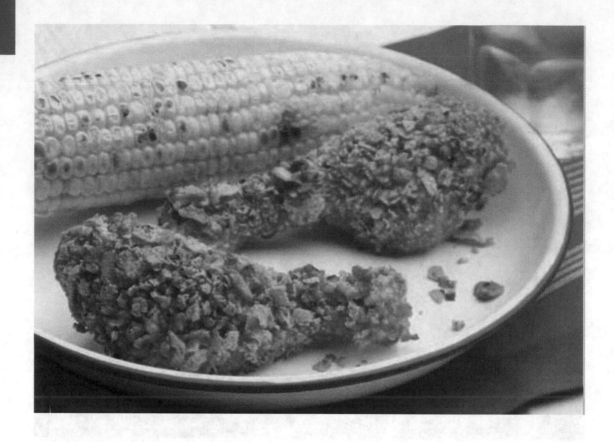

Crispy Oven-Fried Chicken

Ingredients

½ cup fat-free milk or buttermilk
1 tsp poultry seasoning, divided
1 cup cornflakes, crumbled
1½ Tbsp onion powder
1½ Tbsp garlic powder
2 tsp black pepper

2 tsp dried hot pepper, crushed
1 tsp ginger, ground
8 pieces skinless chicken
    (4 breasts, 4 drumsticks)
Paprika, to taste
1 tsp vegetable oil

Steps

1. Add ½ tsp of poultry seasoning to milk.
2. Combine onion powder, garlic powder, black pepper, hot pepper, and ginger with cornflake crumbs; place in large zip-top plastic bag.
3. Wash chicken pieces and pat dry. Dip chicken into milk and shake to remove excess. Place chicken in bag with seasonings and crumbs, and shake quickly.
4. Remove chicken from bag, place on a plate, cover, and refrigerate for 1 hour.
5. Preheat oven to 350°F.
6. Remove chicken from refrigerator, arrange chicken evenly on greased baking pan, and sprinkle lightly with paprika.
7. Cover with aluminum foil and bake for 30 minutes. Remove foil and continue baking for another 10-15 minutes or until meat can easily be pulled away from the bone with fork. Drumsticks may require less baking time than breasts. Crumbs will form crispy "skin." Note: Do not turn chicken during baking.

Yield: 5 servings (1 breast or 4 small drumsticks)
Per serving: 273 calories, 7 g total fat, 2 g sat fat, 39 g protein, 11 g carbs, 1 g fiber, 2 g sugar, 181 mg sodium
Recipe (adapted) and photo: National Heart, Lung & Blood Institute, wecan.nhlbi.NIH.gov

Baked Pork Chops

Ingredients

6 lean center-cut pork chops*, ½-inch thick

1 egg white

1 cup fat-free evaporated milk

¾ cup cornflake crumbs

¼ cup fine, dry breadcrumbs

4 tsp paprika

2 tsp dried oregano

¾ tsp chili powder

2 tsp garlic powder

2 tsp black pepper

⅛ tsp cayenne pepper

⅛ teaspoon dry mustard

½ tsp salt

Nonstick cooking spray, as needed

Steps

1. Preheat oven to 375°F. Trim fat from pork chops.
2. Beat together egg white and fat-free evaporated milk. Place pork chops in milk mixture and let stand for 5 minutes, turning once.
3. Meanwhile, mix cornflake crumbs, breadcrumbs, spices, and salt in small bowl.
4. Use nonstick cooking spray to lightly coat 13x9-inch baking pan.
5. Remove pork chops from milk mixture and coat thoroughly with crumb mixture.
6. Place pork chops on rimmed baking sheet and bake for 20 minutes. Turn pork chops and bake for an additional 15 minutes or until the meat reaches an internal temperature of 145°F. Let the meat rest 3 minutes before serving.

   *This recipe also can be made with skinless, boneless chicken or turkey, or fish; adjust baking times as needed.

Yield: 6 servings (1 chop)

Per serving: 328 calories, 9 g total fat, 3 g sat fat, 46 g protein, 14 g carbs, 1 g fiber, 6 g sugar, 428 mg sodium

Recipe (adapted) and photo: National Heart, Lung & Blood Institute, wecan.nhlbi.nih.gov

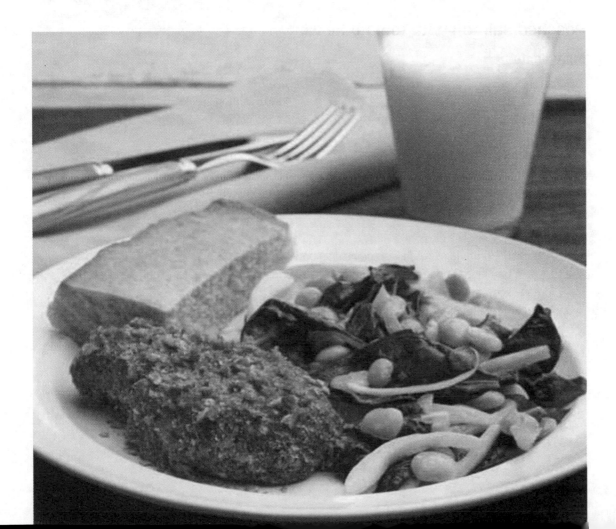

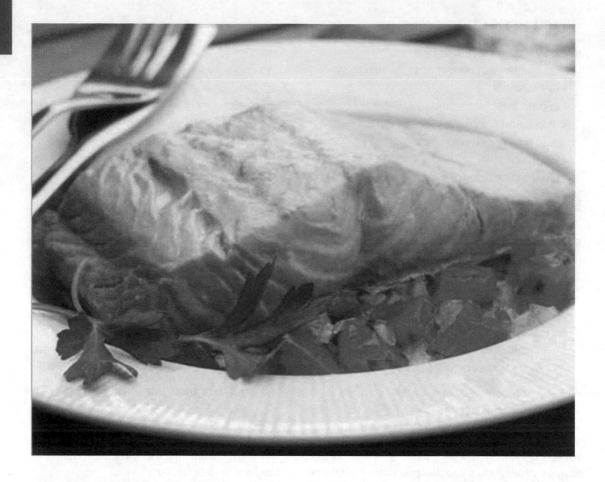

Poached Salmon with Tomato Relish

Ingredients

Relish:
- 2 medium tomatoes, chopped
- 2 Tbsp yellow onion, finely chopped
- 2 Tbsp fresh parsley, finely chopped
- 1 tsp red pepper flakes, or to taste
- ¼ cup red wine vinegar
- 2 Tbsp extra-virgin olive oil
- Black pepper, to taste

Salmon:
- 4 5-oz salmon steaks
- 3 cups water
- 4 black peppercorns
- 1 lemon, thickly sliced
- 3 parsley sprigs
- 1 small onion, thickly sliced
- 2 bay leaves

Steps

1. For relish, combine all relish ingredients in a bowl; set aside.
2. Using a pan large enough to hold salmon steaks, bring water to a boil and add peppercorns, lemon slices, parsley, onion, and bay leaf.
3. Reduce heat and simmer, covered, to let flavors infuse for 5 minutes. Add salmon steaks; make sure they are covered with water. Add additional water if needed.
4. Cook, uncovered, for 10 to 12 minutes or until fish is just tender. It will flake easily when tested with a fork. Never let water boil or fish will toughen.
5. Place one salmon steak on each plate; top each steak with one-quarter of relish.

Yield: 4 servings (1 salmon steak and ¼ cup relish)
Per serving: 354 calories, 23 g total fat, 4 g sat fat, 29 g protein, 7 g carbs, 3 g fiber, 3 g sugar, 92 mg sodium
Recipe (adapted) and photo: National Heart, Lung & Blood Institute, wecan.nhlbi.nih.gov

Easy Peach Crisp

Ingredients

1 Tbsp plus 1 tsp olive oil, divided
½ cup rolled oats
1 tsp sugar
¼ tsp cinnamon
2 cups peaches, diced (or apples, berries, etc.)
Vanilla frozen yogurt (optional)

Steps

1. Preheat oven to 350°F. Grease a 6½-inch cast iron skillet with 1 teaspoon olive oil.
2. In a small bowl, toss oats with cinnamon, sugar, and remaining olive oil.
3. Put fruit in skillet and top with oat mixture. Bake for 35 minutes, until fruit is bubbly and oats are golden brown.
4. Let cool for 5-10 minutes; top with a scoop of vanilla frozen yogurt, if desired. (Caution: skillet will be very hot.)

Yield: 2 servings
Per serving, without yogurt: 209 calories, 11 g total fat, 1 g sat fat, 6 g protein, 34 g carbs, 6 g fiber, 14 g sugar, 1 mg sodium
Recipe (adapted) and photo: Oldways, www.oldwayspt.org

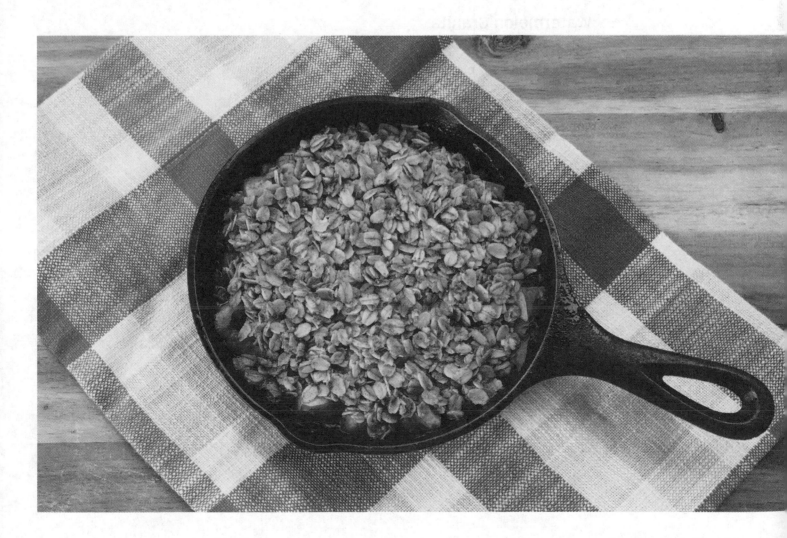

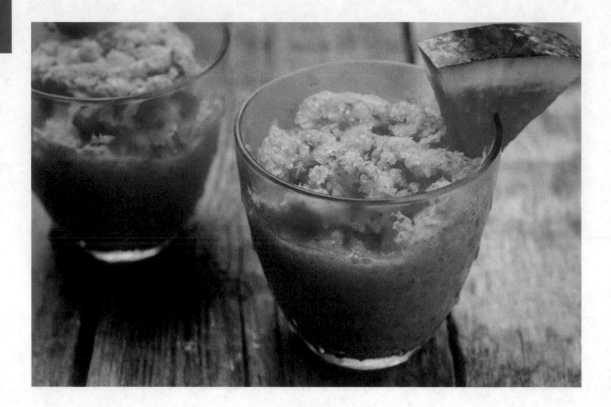

Watermelon Granita

Ingredients:

Zest and juice of 2 medium limes
2 tsp sugar, divided
⅓ cup water
4-5 cups cubed seedless watermelon
Mint leaves for garnish, if desired

Steps

1. In small bowl, combine zest, 1 teaspoon sugar, and lime juice.
2. In small saucepan, combine remaining sugar with ⅓ cup water. Bring mixture to boil. When sugar is dissolved, remove from heat, add zest mixture, stir, and cool to room temperature.
3. In blender or food processor, purée melon to make 3 cups liquid; add lime juice mixture and blend. Pour melon mixture into 9"x 9" metal pan.
4. Cover with plastic wrap and place in freezer. Freeze until slightly hard, 6-8 hours. To serve, scrape melon mixture with fork and scoop mixture into serving bowls. Garnish with mint, if desired.

Yield: 4 (¾-cup) servings
Per serving: 78 calories, 0 g total fat, 0 g sat fat, 1 g protein, 21 g carbs, 2 g fiber, 15 g sugar, 3 mg sodium
Recipe (adapted) and photo: American Institute for Cancer Research, www.aicr.org

Yogurt Pops

Ingredients

6 oz plain, fat-free yogurt
¾ cup 100-percent fruit juice (grape, apple, cherry, orange)

Steps

1. Put the yogurt and juice in a bowl; mix thoroughly. Pour the yogurt mix into 4 small plastic cups (or double the recipe and pour into 8 cups). Put a popsicle stick in the center of each cup.
2. Place the yogurt pops in the freezer until they become solid.

Yield: 4 servings
Per serving: 47 calories, 0 g total fat, 0 g sat fat, 3 g protein, 9 g carbs, 0 g fiber, 7 g sugar, 34 mg sodium
Recipe (adapted): USDA Healthy Eating on a Budget
Photo: © Arinahabich08 | Dreamstime.com

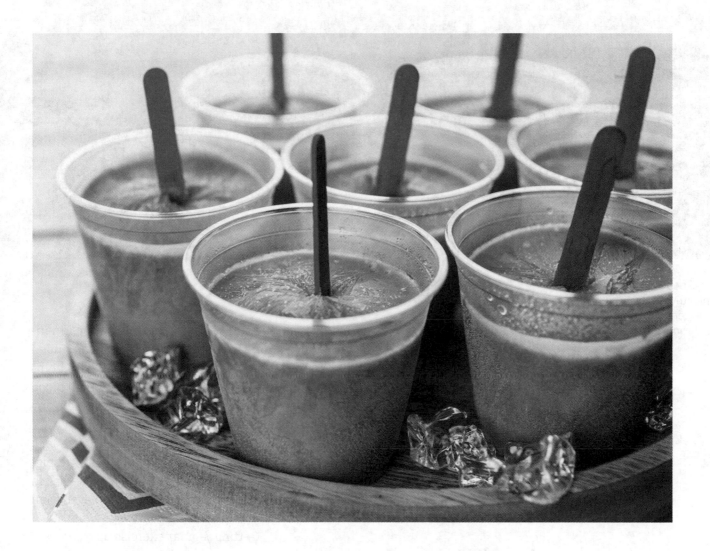

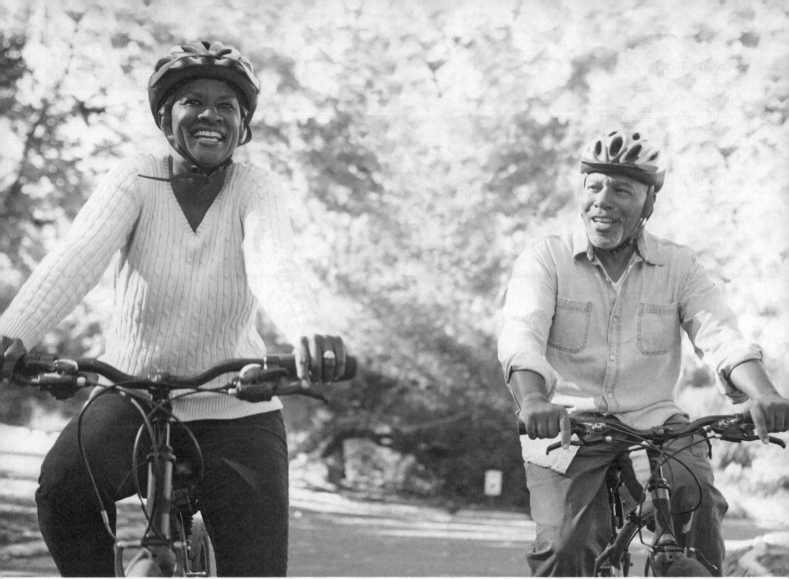

© Monkey Business Images | Dreamstime

Physical activity is a key element in a healthy lifestyle that will help protect your heart and brain from chronic disease.

8 Habits for Heart and Brain Health

The recipes in the previous chapter are a smart way to jump-start healthy eating habits that will benefit your heart and brain. Eating right is only part of the equation, however: Getting plenty of physical activity, sleeping well, and managing your stress level are essential, too. Combined with a healthy dietary pattern, these habits can improve your lodds of avoiding cardiovascular disease and cognitive decline.

Get Moving

You probably already know that exercise is good for your cardiovascular system. Indeed, the scientific evidence that regular physical activity benefits your heart is overwhelming. The latest Physical Activity Guidelines for Americans, updated in late 2018, concluded that, for adults, physical activity helps prevent heart disease, stroke, high blood pressure, and type 2 diabetes, among other conditions.

One study even reported that lack of physical activity was the single biggest contributor to heart-disease risk in women over age 30—more so even than smoking or being overweight.

Getting regular exercise also can help prevent the natural rise in blood pressure that occurs with aging—a key risk factor for stroke. In another study, scientists analyzed the fitness of almost 14,000 men, ages 20 to 60, who did not initially have high blood pressure. After

36 years of follow-up, participants' average blood pressure was found to have risen steadily with age. Men with the lowest fitness level, however, hit an average systolic blood pressure above 120 mmHg eight years earlier than the fittest men.

Exercise for Your Brain

The evidence that physical activity helps protect your brain keeps adding up. The updated physical activity guidelines specifically concluded that exercise reduces the risk of dementia, including Alzheimer's disease.

For example, one study reported that participants who were most physically active were least likely to develop cognitive decline.

More evidence linking physical activity to brain benefits comes from a study of almost 900 older men and women who had complete medical and cognitive tests, answered questionnaires about their physical activity, and underwent MRI scans of their brains. After five years, the most active one-quarter of participants had significantly more gray matter in parts of the brain associated with memory and higher-level thinking than those who with the most sedentary lifestyles. Greater gray-matter volume was associated with a lower risk of developing mild or severe cognitive impairment.

Even people with dementia might benefit from a regular walk, according to a 2018 study. The researchers studied people with vascular dementia who were divided into two groups; one group did a walking program, while the other group (the control group) made no changes in their activity level. After six months, physical and cognitive tests and brain scans showed that people in the walking program had lower blood pressure and showed improvements on the cognitive tests. Brain scans also showed the walkers required less brain activity to maintain attention and make quick decisions than the control group.

Every Minute Helps

Experts recommend that you get at least two-and-a-half hours, or 150 minutes, of moderate exercise every week. Any type of physical activity counts, including a brisk walk, aerobics, swimming, hiking, and doing household chores such as vacuuming or gardening. Previous guidelines that specified activity increments of at least 10 minutes were needed to provide benefits have been modified; the important thing is to get up and get moving, even if it's for two minutes or five minutes. If you have a medical condition, such as arthritis, COPD, or chronic back pain, that makes it difficult to exercise, ask your doctor for a referral to a health-care professional such as a physical therapist who can give you guidance and training in the types of exercise that are appropriate for you.

How you spend your leisure time also matters. According to a Swedish study,

---

Guidelines for Exercise

Updated in November 2018, the *Physical Activity Guidelines for Americans* issued by the U.S. Department of Health and Human Services emphasize that everyone should avoid inactivity. Some physical activity is better than none, and adults who participate in any amount of physical activity gain some health benefits. Specific guidelines for adults include:

- The first key guideline for adults is to move more and sit less. This recommendation is based on new evidence that shows a strong relationship between increased sedentary behavior and increased risk of heart disease, high blood pressure, and all-cause mortality. All physical activity, especially moderate-to-vigorous activity, can help offset these risks.

- To attain the most health benefits from physical activity, adults need at least 150 to 300 minutes of moderate-intensity aerobic activity, like brisk walking or fast dancing, each week. Adults also need muscle-strengthening activity, like lifting weights or doing push-ups, at least two days each week.

- When older adults cannot do 150 minutes of moderate-intensity aerobic activity a week because of chronic conditions, they should be as physically active as their abilities and conditions allow.

- The previous guidelines stated that only 10-minute bouts of physical activity counted toward meeting the guidelines. This requirement has been removed because all activity counts.

- There are immediate health benefits, attainable from a single bout of activity, including reduced anxiety and blood pressure, improved quality of sleep, and improved insulin sensitivity.

There are more long-term benefits from physical activity, including improved brain health, reduced risk of eight types of cancer (previously two), reduced risk for fall-related injuries in older adults, and reduced risk of excessive weight gain.

Activity Boosts "Cognitive Reserve"

Even in people with brain lesions or biomarkers of dementia, higher levels of physical activity can help protect cognitive function. That's the conclusion of a post-mortem study of 454 people with an average age at death of 91; 191 participants had been diagnosed with dementia. Researchers administered 10 motor-performance tests using accelerometers about two years before participants died. Participants with higher levels of physical activity and motor ability had better cognition, regardless of what subsequent study found in their brains. There was no evidence, however, that physical activity directly protected cognition against dementia pathologies. Instead, scientists posited that an active lifestyle contributes to a "cognitive reserve" that helps maintain function independent of accumulating brain pathologies. They wrote, "The results of randomized trials of physical exercise suggest that exercise leads to increases in brain tissue, including in the hippocampus, where atrophy is an early and important finding in Alzheimer's disease."

Neurology, Feb. 19, 2019

adults participating in active leisure (yard work, home repairs, bicycling) were at 30 percent lower risk for all-cause mortality and 27 percent lower risk for a first-time cardiovascular event compared to those who spent their leisure time sitting in front of a television or a computer.

The Importance of Sleep

Getting a good night's rest is also important to your heart and brain. People who otherwise adhere to a healthy lifestyle and who also sleep at least seven hours a night have been shown to be less likely to suffer cardiovascular disease. Good sleepers are less likely to die from cardiovascular causes than those with otherwise healthy lifestyles who don't get adequate sleep.

Poor sleep quality and diet may contribute to the early accumulation of the plaques associated with Alzheimer's disease, according to a review of the scientific evidence. Part of the reason may involve cortisol, a hormone that plays a role in regulating many core functions, including sleep. Cortisol levels naturally rise and fall with day and night, but diets high in refined sugars, salt, animal fats, and animal proteins and low in fruits and vegetables can disrupt the circadian levels of cortisol, leading to poor sleep quality. Dietary changes that influence the body's cortisol levels—and in turn promote good sleep—might be a safe and novel way to help protect the brain, scientists suggest. The review also notes that, independent of diet, sleep disorders and poor sleep quality are associated with a higher risk of Alzheimer's disease.

A good night's sleep seems to be important for the brain to clear the beta-amyloids that form the plaques associated with Alzheimer's disease. In another study, researchers demonstrated that disrupted sleep may help explain how those beta-amyloid proteins begin to damage the brain: The less deep sleep

participants got, the higher the amount of beta-amyloid in their brains, and the more words in a memory test they forgot overnight.

Findings from several other studies suggest sleeping too little or too much, abnormal breathing during sleep, and excessive daytime sleepiness are associated with a higher risk of cognitive impairment.

Too much sleep may be as much of an issue as too little, however. In a long-running study, women who slept either two hours more or less than seven hours per night scored lower on cognitive tests than women who slept about seven hours per night. Those sleeping five hours or less and nine hours or more also had beta-amyloid markers in their blood that predicted a greater risk of cognitive decline and dementia.

Ways to Improve Sleep

A good start on getting better, more restful sleep is to improve your sleep environment and "sleep hygiene." Here are some tips:

- Eat dinner or any snacks at least three hours before bedtime.
- Avoid caffeine (soda, tea, coffee) within several hours of bedtime.
- Get into a regular sleep routine. Go to bed at about the same time each night and wake up at about the same time each morning, even on weekends.
- Relax before bed by soaking in a warm tub, reading, or listening to calming music.
- Keep your bedroom cool, quiet, and dark.
- Avoid activities on a computer, cell phone, or tablet for at least an hour prior to bedtime; mental activity, as well as the light from electronic devices, can disturb your sleep-wake pattern.

After trying these strategies, if you still have problems sleeping and often feel tired during the day, report it to your doctor and discuss possible causes and solutions. If your doctor is unable to identify the reasons for your poor sleep, he or she may refer you to a doctor who specializes in sleep disorders.

Risks from Tobacco

Smoking, which sharply increases your risks of lung disease and cancer, also damages your heart and brain. Smoking increases your risk of high blood pressure, heart disease, and stroke. One review of the evidence regarding smoking and cognitive function concluded that smoking is a significant risk factor for Alzheimer's disease.

The good news for smokers is that it's never too late to quit. Within 20 minutes after stubbing out that last cigarette, your heart rate and blood pressure will drop. In just two weeks, your circulation will improve, and. within a year, your coronary heart disease risk will drop to half of what it was when you smoked.

For tools and tips to help you quit, see smokefree.gov.

Stress Affects Heart and Brain

When you're stressed, your body releases chemicals, such as cortisol and norepinephrine, that quicken your heartbeat and breathing and put your body into a state of alert. In the short term, these effects aren't harmful. When stress is chronic, however, the ongoing release of these chemicals can affect your immune system and make you more vulnerable to health problems. Chronic stress can be bad for both your heart and your brain.

In your brain, when you are in stressful situations over which you feel you have no control, an enzyme called protein kinase C ("PKC") is activated. This enzyme affects the brain's prefrontal cortex, which regulates thought, behavior, and emotion. Too much PKC can impair your ability to concentrate, leading to distractibility and impaired judgment.

Try these strategies to lower your stress level:

- **Get moving.** Physical activity releases chemicals called endorphins, which have effects similar to morphine, including a reduced perception of pain and a feeling of well-being.
- **Try deep breathing,** meditation, or yoga. There are many variations of these relaxation techniques; explore options until you find one that is well-suited for you.
- **Take a mental "break."** Sit quietly, close your eyes, breathe deeply, and visualize yourself in a peaceful, relaxing place.
- **Have a good laugh.** Laughter can help reduce your blood pressure and stress hormone levels.
- **Start a stress journal.** Keeping track of stressors and your responses to them can help you control how you react to stress.

It's Up to You

Together with a healthy dietary pattern, these lifestyle changes can go a long way toward reducing your risk of heart disease and cognitive decline. You now know which dietary patterns are recommended by nutrition experts, as well as the foods and nutrients that support the optimal functioning of your brain and heart.

While lifestyle choices can't completely protect you against cardiovascular disease or cognitive decline and dementia, following a healthy diet and making other changes represent the best steps current science can offer.

The human heart may not really be "the root of all faculties" as people once believed, but the connection between heart and brain is essential to your well-being. By making smart choices, your journey to better heart and brain health can start today.

Alzheimer's disease: A progressive, irreversible and incurable form of dementia due to deterioration of brain tissue. It leads to memory loss, personality changes, and other mental impairment. It is the most common form of dementia and it affects an estimated 5.4 million people in the U.S. (See: Dementia)

antioxidants: A substance in the blood that protect cells from damage caused by harmful unstable molecules produced in response to stress or exposure to environmental toxins. Antioxidants include flavonoids, beta-carotene, lycopene, selenium, and vitamins A, C, and E. Many more compounds in fruits, vegetables, legumes, nuts, and whole grains are antioxidants.

arrhythmia: An irregular heart rate in which the heart beats too slowly, too quickly, or out of its normal rhythm. Some arrhythmias aren't serious, while others are life-threatening.

artery: A major blood vessel that supplies oxygen-rich blood to the body's tissues. Arteries can become clogged with plaque, which blocks blood flow and can increase the risks for a heart attack or stroke.

atherosclerosis: A disease characterized by enlarging deposits (called plaques) of certain fats (including cholesterol), calcium and blood clots on the inside surface of arteries. As the deposits grow, they can severely restrict or block the flow of blood. Atherosclerosis in the coronary arteries is called coronary artery disease (CAD). Inflammation in the plaques can lead to their disruption, the formation of clots in the coronaries and heart attacks.

body mass index (BMI): A calculation that combines weight and height: (Weight in Pounds / [Height in inches x Height in inches]) x 703. A BMI of over 25 is considered overweight, and over 30 is obese.

carotid artery disease: Narrowing of the major blood vessel in the neck that supplies the brain with oxygen-rich blood. It is caused by the buildup of plaque inside the artery walls.

cholesterol: A waxy, fat-like substance found in foods of animal origin and synthesized by the body that can contribute to arteriosclerosis ("hardening of the arteries"), but that is secondary to saturated fat. In the blood, serum cholesterol combines with proteins to form LDL and HDL cholesterol. In large amounts in the blood, cholesterol can clog arteries.

cognition: Conscious intellectual activity, such as thinking and memory, orientation, language, judgment, and problem-solving.

cognitive decline: A loss of cognitive function, such as that associated with dementia.

coronary artery disease (CAD): A condition caused by the buildup of fatty plaques in the artery walls, which narrows the blood vessels and prevents enough oxygen from reaching the heart. CAD is the most common type of heart disease and the leading cause of death in the U.S. in both men and women.

dementia: A progressive illness that results in memory loss and other cognitive abnormalities that over time seriously interfere with daily life. There are several forms of dementia, the most common of which is Alzheimer's diseasese.

heart attack: Injury or death of some of the heart muscle, usually caused by a blood clot. Heart attack is also known as myocardial infarction (MI).

heart failure (congestive heart failure, CHF): A chronic, progressive disease in which the heart muscle weakens and can no longer pump blood well enough to meet the body's needs.

hemorrhagic stroke: A stroke caused by a weakened blood vessel in the brain that ruptures and bleeds.

high-density lipoprotein (HDL) cholesterol: Often referred to as "good" cholesterol, HDL cholesterol reduces cholesterol buildup in the arteries, thereby reducing the risk of heart disease. (See also: Cholesterol, low-density lipoprotein [LDL] cholesterol).

hypertension: High blood pressure. Known as "the silent killer," hypertension is a very important risk factor for stroke and heart attack as well as other disorders.

ischemic stroke: A stroke caused when a blood clot develops in an artery in the brain or a blood clot travels to the brain from another location.

low-density lipoprotein (LDL) cholesterol: Often referred to as "bad" cholesterol, LDL cholesterol is a fatty substance that can build up in the arteries and lead to cardiovascular disease. LDL contains more fat and less protein than HDL.

mild cognitive impairment (MCI): A stage between normal forgetfulness due to aging and more serious cognitive decline.

omega-3 fatty acids: Essential fatty acids found in fish, walnuts, soy products, and some seeds and vegetable oils that can reduce the risk of cardiovascular disease and improve brain function.

omega-6 fatty acids: A type of unsaturated fat found in many nuts, seeds, and vegetable oils, and in some poultry, seafood, and vegetables. One omega-6 fatty acid, linoleic acid, is essential to the body.

phytochemicals (also called phytonutrients): Compounds in plants that provide flavor, aroma, and color, and protect the plant from microbes and environmental damage. When consumed by humans, phytochemicals are believed to promote health and prevent disease. Many phytochemicals have antioxidant properties.

saturated fat: A type of fat that can increase unhealthy cholesterol levels and raise the risk of heart disease. Saturated fatty acids are found primarily in animal foods, especially meats and full-fat dairy products.

stroke: An acute vascular event that occurs in the brain. It is most often caused by a blood clot that lodges in an artery and blocks the flow of blood to the brain (ischemic stroke), producing symptoms ranging from paralysis of limbs and loss of speech to unconsciousness and death. Less commonly, a stroke may be caused by bleeding into the brain (hemorrhagic stroke).

trans fat (or trans fatty acid): A type of fat that is manufactured by adding hydrogen to liquid oil to solidify it, resulting in the formation of a partially hydrogenated oil. Trans fat increases unhealthy LDL cholesterol levels and lowers healthy HDL cholesterol levels. Note: The clear evidence of its harmful health effects resulted in a ban on trans fat by the U.S. Food & Drug Administration.

unsaturated fat: A type of fatty acid that lowers cholesterol levels and reduces the risk for coronary artery disease when it is consumed in place of saturated and trans fats. Monounsaturated and polyunsaturated fatty acids fall into this category.

vascular dementia: Dementia caused by blood vessel damage in the brain, the second-most-common form of dementia after Alzheimer's disease ease.

whole grains: Grains that contain all the essential parts and naturally occurring nutrients of the entire grain seed—the bran, germ, and endosperm.

Academy of Nutrition and Dietetics
eatright.org
800-877-1600
120 S. Riverside Plaza, Suite 2190
Chicago, IL 60606-6995

Alzheimer's Association
www.alz.org
800-272-3900 (24/7 helpline)
312-335-8700
225 N. Michigan Ave.
Chicago, IL 60611-7633

American Heart Association
www.heart.org
800-242-8721
7272 Greenville Ave.
Dallas, TX 75231

American Institute for Cancer Research
aicr.org
800-843-8114
1560 Wilson Blvd., Suite 1000
Arlington, VA 22209

Centers for Disease Control and Prevention (CDC)
cdc.gov
800-232-4636
1600 Clifton Rd.
Atlanta, GA 30329-4027

Food and Drug Administration
www.fda.gov
888-463-6332
10903 New Hampshire Ave.
Silver Spring, MD 20993

Friedman School of Nutrition Science and Policy—Tufts University
nutrition.tufts.edu
617-636-3737
150 Harrison Ave.
Boston, MA 02111

Jean Mayer USDA Human Nutrition Research Center of Aging
hnrca.tufts.edu
617-556-3000
711 Washington St.
Boston, MA 02111

National Institutes of Health
nih.gov
301-496-4000
9000 Rockville Pike
Bethesda, MD 20892

National Heart, Lung and Blood Institute (NHLBI)
www.nhlbi.nih.gov
Bldg 31
3131 Center Dr.
Bethesda, MD 20892

Oldways Whole Grains Council
wholegrainscouncil.org
617-421-5500
266 Beacon St.
Boston, MA 02116

Tufts University *Health & Nutrition Letter*
www.nutritionletter.tufts.edu
PO Box 5656
Norwalk, CT 06856

Tufts' MyPlate for Older Adults
hnrca.tufts.edu/myplate

U.S. Department of Agriculture Center for Nutrition Policy and Promotion
cnpp.usda.gov
ChooseMyPlate.gov
202-720-2791
3101 Park Center Dr. 10th Fl.
Alexandria, VA 22302-1594

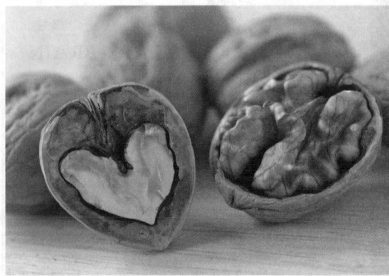
© Calypsoart | Dreamstime

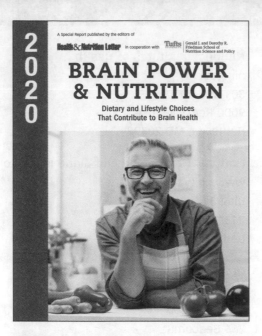
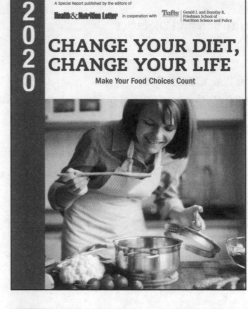
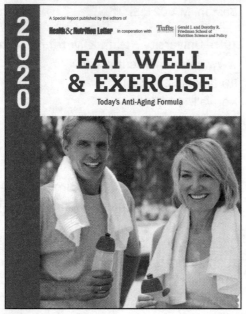
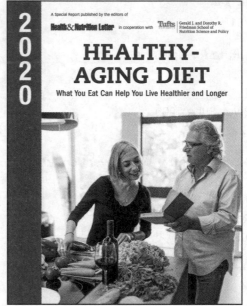
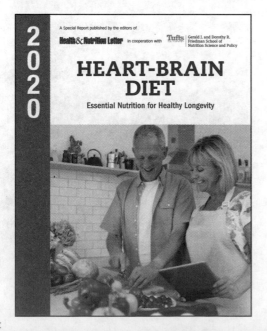